FIX YOUR GENES to FIT YOUR JEANS

Optimizing diet, health and weight through personal genetics

Dr. Penny Kendall-Reed BSc ND
Naturopathic Doctor

Dr. Stephen Reed BM BCh MA MSc FRCSC
Orthopaedic Surgeon

Fix Your Genes to Fit Your Jeans
Copyright © 2020 by Penny Kendall-Reed

All rights reserved. No part of this publication may be reproduced, distributed, or transmitted in any form or by any means, including photocopying, recording, or other electronic or mechanical methods, without the prior written permission of the author, except in the case of brief quotations embodied in critical reviews and certain other non-commercial uses permitted by copyright law.

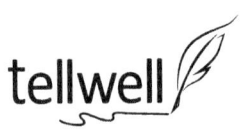

Tellwell Talent
www.tellwell.ca

ISBN
978-0-2288-2903-4 (Hardcover)
978-0-2288-2902-7 (Paperback)
978-0-2288-2904-1 (eBook)

Disclaimer

This book is not intended as a substitute for the medical advice of physicians. The reader should regularly consult a physician in matters relating to his/her health and particularly with respect to any symptoms that may require diagnosis or medical attention. The information provided in this book is designed to provide guidance on the subjects discussed. This book is not meant to be used, nor should it be used, to diagnose or treat any medical condition. For diagnosis or treatment of any medical problem, consult your own physician. Nutritional supplements are included in treatment protocols but are not essential. It is highly recommended that before starting any supplement program, you discuss them with your health-care practitioner. The publisher and authors are not responsible for any specific health or allergy needs that may require medical supervision and are not liable for any damages or negative consequences from any treatment, action, application or preparation, to any person reading or following the information in this book. References are provided for informational purposes only and do not constitute endorsement of any websites or other sources. Readers should be aware that the websites listed in this book may change. Any products included in this book are offered as suggestions and do not constitute definitive therapy. Manufacturers of these products have no involvement or responsibility relating to this book.

TABLE OF CONTENTS

Chapter 1	Introduction: Why You Need to Read This Book	1
Chapter 2	Case Study #1	13
Chapter 3	DNA, Genes and SNPs (Single Nucleotide Polymorphisms)	17
Chapter 4	SNPs, Disease and Epigenetics	46
Chapter 5	Case Study #2	69
Chapter 6	Which Genes, Which SNPs?	72
Chapter 7	Case Study # 3	86
Chapter 8	FTO	90
Chapter 9	ADIPOQ	112
Chapter 10	MC4R	123
Chapter 11	PPARG	132
Chapter 12	APOA2	144
Chapter 13	FABP2	150
Chapter 14	TCF7L2	161
Chapter 15	IRS1	169
Chapter 16	Case Study #4	179
Chapter 17	The Stress Genes	182
Chapter 18	Case Study #5	200
Chapter 19	Proteins, Fats and Carbohydrates	204
Chapter 20	Meal Timing and Intermittent Fasting	223
Chapter 21	Case Study #6	233
Chapter 22	Conclusion	236
Appendix 1	Food Tables	239
Appendix 2	Supplements	248
Appendix 3	Resources	256
Glossary of Terms		259
References		271
About the Authors		301

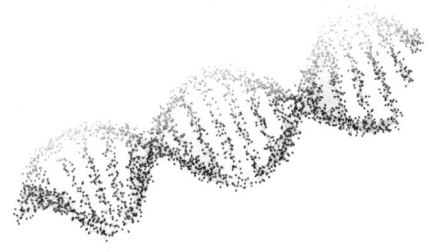

CHAPTER 1
Introduction: Why You Need to Read This Book

How Your Genes Affect Your Health and Metabolism and Determine Your Ideal Diet

We used to think there was little we could do about the genes we'd been given. They were carved in stone and we were at the mercy of their bidding. It was a fatalistic attitude often used as an excuse to avoid making changes to our lives. What was the point if our genes were immutable?

Well, it turns out that we were wrong! Although it is true that we cannot change our genetic code, we *can* greatly influence the expression of many genes and control the effects they have on our body. By making small changes to our lifestyle, our diet and our supplements, we can optimize the genetic blueprint we have been given and even alter the way genes work. We can turn them on or off, up or down to maximize their beneficial side, while minimizing their adverse effects. We can steer them in a specific direction that enhances our health today and we can modify them to prevent problems in the future. Genes, it would appear, are malleable, and with the right tools we can shape them to create better health and longevity.

When I started clinical practice in 1996, I rapidly realized that although the knowledge and training gained from my years as a student were comprehensive, they did not explain the idiosyncrasies of individual patients. Diagnosis and patterns of treatment were useful in many cases, but as I delved deeper into the complexities of metabolic health, I found I needed to expand my spectrum of management. My research took me through numerous dietary trends, supplement regimens and lifestyle modifications. I explored a variety of different nutritional programs and "fad" diets, even producing two of my own, *The New Naturopathic Diet* (Winding Star Press, 2002, ISBN: 1 55082 302 7) and *The No Crave Diet* (Virgin Books, 2008, ISBN: 978 0 7535 1313 2). The number of available diets has since exploded, offering a bewildering array of options for the health- and weight-conscious consumer. A summary of the more popular diets is given below.

Summary of Popular Diets

The Atkins Diet
- *High-protein, high-fat, low-carbohydrate diet*
- *Created by cardiologist Robert Atkins in 1972 and republished in 1992*
- *Initial "ketogenic" phase with carbohydrates limited to 20 grams per day. Fat and protein intake are unlimited. The body switches to using fat as a fuel source*
- *Subsequent phases allow gradually reintroduction of carbohydrates until the individual establishes their "critical carbohydrate level" for stable weight*
- *More recent versions such as Atkins 20 and 40 allow higher carbohydrate intake and recommend healthier fat and protein choices*

The South Beach Diet
- *High-protein, low-fat, low-carbohydrate diet*
- *Designed by cardiologist Dr. Agatston and published in 2003*

- *Phase 1 eliminates simple sugars, grains, starches, fruits, sweets and processed foods, while encouraging high protein, low fat and unlimited vegetables*
- *Phase 2 allows the reintroduction of limited fruits and grains*
- *Phase 3 recommends following Phase 2 guidelines but in a more relaxed fashion*

Vegan Diets
- *Lifestyle plant-based diet with no restrictions on macronutrients*
- *Consists only of plant-based foods such as vegetables, grains, nuts and fruits*
- *No animal products including dairy and eggs*
- *Five portions of fruits and vegetables per day recommended*
- *Main meals should include potatoes, bread, rice or pasta*
- *Dairy alternatives include soy drinks or soy yoghurts*
- *Beans and pulses are encouraged as the main source of protein*

Ketogenic Diets
- *Very-low-carbohydrate (5%), high-fat (75%), moderate-protein (20%) diet*
- *Even healthy carbohydrates such as vegetables are very limited*
- *Similar to Atkins in that it forces the body to switch to starvation mode using fat as the primary fuel source*
- *Standard and high-protein versions do not reintroduce carbohydrates*
- *Cyclical and Targeted versions allow carbohydrates intermittently*
- *Includes versions such as The Bulletproof Diet*

The Zone Diet
- 40% complex carbohydrates, 30% unsaturated fat, 30% lean protein
- Designed by biochemist Dr. Barry Sears and published in 1995
- Designed to reduce inflammation
- Meal size includes 1/3 plate-size lean protein, 2/3 carbohydrates and minimal fat
- All food is to be consumed at three meals and two snacks

The Dukan Diet
- High-protein, low-carbohydrate diet
- Adds oat bran for satiety and to reduce fat absorption
- Developed by French physician Dr. Pierre Dukan and published in 2000
- Phase 1 (Attack Stage) is essentially protein plus oat bran
- Phase 2 (Cruise Phase) allows minimal complex carbohydrates
- Subsequent phases reintroduce more carbohydrates
- Long-term Stabilization Phase is predominantly high protein, low carbohydrate with increased oat bran

The Pritikin Diet
- Very-low-fat, high-fibre diet with emphasis on the calorie density of foods
- Designed by Robert Pritikin and published in 1979
- Stresses the importance of exercise
- Similar to Vegan Diets in that plant-based foods are the main focus
- Fish and small amounts of lean protein allowed
- Low in fat and refined carbohydrates

> *Fasting diets in which meal timing is altered to include periods of fasting or calorie restriction*
> - *Calorie Restriction (CR) – an ongoing reduction in caloric intake without malnutrition*
> - *Intermittent Fasting (I.F.) – fasting for 12 to 16 hours on a daily basis*
> - *Time Restricted Feeding (TRF) – eating only within a specific 8- to 12-hour period of the day*
> - *Alternate Day Fasting (ADF) – no calories are consumed on fasting days with unrestricted food intake on "feast" days*
> - *Alternate Day Modified Fasting (ADMF) – similar to TRF but with 25% of the baseline energy needed on "fasting" days alternated with unrestricted food intake on "feast" days*
> - *Periodic Fasting (PF) – fasting only one or two days a week and consuming unrestricted food on five or six days per week*
> - *Fasting Mimicking Diet (FMD) – This five-day fasting pattern involves lowering caloric intake to 700 calories per day, with a significant reduction in protein and sugars, and no saturated fats to mimic a fasting response in the body. The five-day fast is completed once every three months*
>
> *(For more information on Intermittent Fasting, see Chapter 20.)*

My patients tried many of these diets, and they worked well for some and not for others. Some patients reported finding a particular diet easy to follow but failed to achieve their goals. Others had success with their health or weight but found the diet impossible to stick to. It seemed that no one diet was the answer for everyone.

I explored the impact of exercise, the environment and chronic stress, and I tried my best to fit patients into diagnostic and therapeutic "boxes" within which I could expect them to improve their health, lose weight and reverse or prevent metabolic parameters such as high blood sugar or cholesterol. It worked well but I found I had to continually expand the number of "boxes" to accommodate everyone. Certain patients did well with some aspects of their treatment but not others, while other patients seemed to require the interaction of two or more boxes. A few failed to fit into any box at all, leaving me in somewhat of a quandary as how to best manage them despite staying on top of current research.

Starting around 2011, I noticed an increasing number of articles referencing individual areas of genetic variation called SNPs, pronounced "snips" and short for Single Nucleotide Polymorphisms. Individual differences in these SNPs are called "alleles" and these alleles provide the basis of your personal genetic coding results from DNA testing. Articles discussed the association of SNP alleles with metabolic function, weight management and the risk of disease, particularly diabetes. So, although SNPs had been recognized for many years as components of our genetic makeup, the emergence of numerous studies examining the correlation of SNP variants with disease risk made them relevant to my practice. The potential to improve diagnostic accuracy, more clearly define risk and hone my therapeutic regimens according to individual genetics was exciting and, in terms of naturopathic medicine, somewhat of a Holy Grail for personalized health.

I began to build my own database of research, focused on SNPs that were both relevant to my patient population and available on different genetic platforms. A "platform" refers to the genetic testing company such as 23andMe and to resources that allow interpretation of SNP results. Early on, these platforms emphasized ethnic origins and major disease risk rather than modifiable parameters. Were you related to Vikings and did you have the BRCA-1 gene (breast cancer risk factor) or how do you handle carbohydrates and fats and what could you do to minimize metabolic disease risk such as diabetes? However, as interest grew, costs fell and the availability of the tests became more widespread, metabolic SNP analysis became an integral component of many platforms. These SNPs were now included in both the genetic sequencing and through the decoders that took raw genetic data and produced a report based on your personal SNP coding. Now, rather than just announcing that you had an "at-risk" coding for a certain gene, platforms began to introduce brief discussions of what this meant in terms of metabolism and physiology along with advice on how one should modify lifestyle in order to account for such genetic idiosyncrasies.

At this point, I ran myself through a number of commercially available genetic tests to see what genes were analyzed and how well the results correlated with what I knew about my personal health. I found that while some of the information was both useful and accurate, many of the genes I knew to be important from my research either were not sequenced or were documented but not analyzed. As my research base developed in concert with the ever-expanding literature, I was able to start formulating programs based on individual SNP patterns. I began to realize why certain patients did not fit into some of the therapeutic "boxes" I had assigned them to and why treatment options that worked for some individuals failed in others that on the surface appeared clinically similar.

As increasing numbers of patients both presented with their genetic analysis or elected to complete it having consulted with me, I recognized that this truly was the next exciting frontier of medicine. Patients were unique and did not fit into pre-designed boxes. As I went over their results, explaining why they felt a certain way after different foods, with varying types of exercise and when stressed or losing sleep, their eyes lit up with a recognition that I truly understood them and their individual issues. "Yes, that's me" would be a common expression at the end of our discussion. I would receive emails a few weeks later from patients seeing improvements in their health, their energy, their sleep and their weight, problems they had struggled with for years without an answer. Patients for whom I had scratched my head trying to figure out why my protocols were not working were suddenly doing amazingly well with simple SNP-based tweaks to their treatment.

Despite this initial success, I was still questioning certain aspects of the analysis and decoding. To a certain degree, patients were still being categorized into boxes, although the boxes were now assigned according to certain individual SNPs rather than based on clinical history and physical examination. Assigning treatment based on one SNP seemed oversimplified, particularly considering the tremendous number of SNPs influencing certain aspects of health and metabolism. There were well-documented interactions between SNPs, and as my database grew, I recognized that patients with a certain SNP profile responded differently dependent on their coding for other complementary SNPs. In addition, available decoders did not take into account the role of epigenetics, the term used to explain the influence factors such as diet, stress and the environment have on whether or not a gene is expressed (active). Incorporating these modifiers into my genetic interpretation and therapeutic protocol design has been the major focus of my research and clinical work for the past five years. Personal genetic testing has the potential to finally offer truly individualized health advice and treatment recommendations.

Personal Genetic Testing

The number of people ordering commercially available DNA tests is going up exponentially. In 2014 there were approximately one million tests ordered worldwide. By 2019 this number was above 25 million with over 90% of tests being performed by Ancestry and 23andMe. Individuals submit a spit sample or cheek swab to the company, which then runs the analysis and provides a report of varying content and complexity. Some are more focussed on heritage and geographic origin, while others advise on different aspects of health including disease risk, nutrition and exercise.

> **Popular Direct-to-Consumer DNA Testing Companies** *(see Appendix 3 for website details)*
>
> Heritage and Origin
> - Ancestry DNA
> - Living DNA
> - My Heritage DNA
>
> Health and Fitness
> - 23andMe
> - ORIG3N
> - HomeDNA
> - CRI genetics
> - Fitness Genes

The accuracy of these tests appears excellent with regard to the health genes but there is some inconsistency as it relates to heritage and geographic origin, which results from variability in company databases. Platforms differ primarily in terms of the genes they test and the advice provided. The question is whether people are using these tests effectively to improve their health. From my experience, patients often present with their genetic data, confused by the report and uncertain how to address many of the health issues they are now aware of.

I have encountered a number of issues that make many reports difficult or unhelpful when it comes to using your genetic data to make useful lifestyle improvements. Some use too many SNPs for the same gene. For example, there are over 100 variations of the metabolic gene FTO, yet only two or three are relevant and clinically supported. Reports also often list numerous genetic variants without any clear explanation of what these mean to your health. Other reports don't use enough SNPs when analyzing a certain metabolic category. For example, they use only one gene to determine carbohydrate tolerance, while an accurate assessment needs to use at least two.

Many reports will tell you that you have a certain SNP coding, along with a very brief explanation of what that means. Unfortunately, those one-line descriptions are often confusing and seem to overlap with other genes. They also rarely offer a comprehensive and easy-to-understand treatment protocol including a clear description of diet, exercise and supplements. You know you're at risk but have no idea what to do about it!

Almost no reports offer comprehensive integrative gene therapy. They look at single genes to make recommendations rather than combinations of genes. One SNP may say "you handle carbs well" while another says "avoid too many carbs," leaving the individual confused and uncertain how to change their lifestyle. ("Carbs" is a common abbreviation for "carbohydrates".)

In this book, my aim is to provide practical and usable information with comprehensive and easy-to-follow treatment options that make sense according to your genetic data.

It is clear to me that our health, metabolism and weight are controlled by the interplay between nature and nurture—between our genetics and our environment. We can now identify our individual genetic strengths and weaknesses through SNP analysis and we can modify our environment through diet, supplements and lifestyle. This gives us the unprecedented ability to influence the way our bodies function, maximizing our health and reducing our propensity for metabolic disease. Our genes can tell us our most favourable balance of macronutrients (protein, fat and carbohydrate) for optimum health and weight management and the ideal number and timing of meals.

I have incorporated my research into an online program called **GeneRx.ca** that coverts the raw genetic SNP data provided by 23andMe into a usable and relevant personalized health report and treatment protocol. The program includes extensive SNP interaction formulae that recognize the interplay between different genes in determining overall function in an individual. It also incorporates analysis and treatment of numerous epigenetic factors including chronic stress, lack of sleep, age and carbohydrate or fat intake. The report covers numerous aspects of individual health, including diet and metabolism and is available to registered health-care professionals and personal trainers for use with their patients and clients. Further details are available at the end of Chapter 6 and on the website *GeneRx.ca*.

This book provides the background to my research over the past 10 years. It explains what SNPs are; how they affect your diet, metabolism and health; and how your lifestyle influences their expression. It allows you to better understand the genetic data you receive from commercially available platforms such as 23andMe. In addition, I have chosen several SNPs that I have found to be the most important when treating my patients and given them detailed explanations along with comprehensive therapeutic protocols. Whether you wish to simply improve your health and eat according to your genes or wish to optimize your weight and reduce the risk of metabolism-associated conditions, this book will provide important answers and guidelines to help you achieve your goals. For individuals planning to start any type of diet, this book provides essential information on how you can use your genetic profile to choose the right one for you.

The five cornerstones of health in my practice are metabolism, diet, stress, inflammation and detoxification. Optimizing these is the foundation of good health and the reduction of disease risk. In this book, we will be looking at genes and SNPs that impact your metabolism, diet and stress. These three factors are closely interlinked when it comes to your weight, energy levels and diet. Some of them are associated with the development of diseases such as type 2 diabetes, but it is important to bear in mind that such diseases have multiple etiologies and contributing factors. So, while you may have a "risk allele," you may never develop the condition. The purpose of the information in this book is simply to identify your own personal strengths and weaknesses and to allow you to make sensible lifestyle choices to potentially improve your overall health and well-being. It may also help you achieve your ideal weight. If it can help reduce your risk for certain diseases, then that is an added benefit.

I understand that there are many factors that influence weight, metabolism and metabolic disease. The etiology of weight gain, metabolic syndrome, type 2 diabetes, heart disease and dyslipidemia (high cholesterol) is complex and multi-faceted, meaning there is no single answer to treatment. I feel that genetics provides another important piece to the puzzle and one that has the potential to be highly individualized.

Note to Readers

This book is designed for a wide audience and contains information that would be of interest and benefit to everyone from a nutritional novice to a health-care practitioner experienced in dietary and metabolic management. As such, certain sections contain more detailed genetic and food-related information. However, understanding all these principles is not essential, and readers will still benefit greatly from this book by using the easy-to-follow advice in the gene and nutrition chapters. Referencing the glossary and some of the chapter summaries will help fill in any gaps.

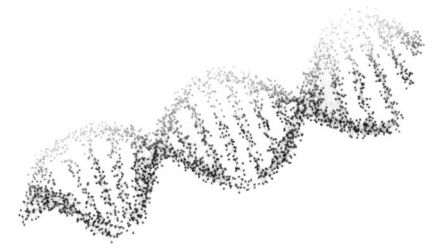

CHAPTER 2
Case Study #1
Using Genetics to Improve Diet and Weight

Anna is a 36-year-old professional woman who came to see me because of unwanted weight gain, despite her strict diet and exercise regimen. Her weight had increased 18 pounds in eight months. She felt hungry all the time, had low energy and had muscle and joint soreness.

Anna had originally wanted to eat more healthily and planned to lose about five pounds. On the recommendation of a friend, she had radically changed her diet from a higher protein, moderate-carbohydrate diet with "minimal fats" to more of a "ketogenic" diet incorporating high fat, low to moderate protein, and restricted carbohydrates with fewer vegetables and no fruits, whole grains or starches.

Within a couple of months of starting the diet, she began to feel "puffy" and inflamed and then started to put on weight. To counteract this, she increased her exercise, running 30 minutes to one hour four times a week, and became stricter with her diet. Despite this, she reported increased feelings of hunger and craving and continued to gain weight. She felt progressively more fatigued, particularly during exercise.

Prior to our initial consultation, Anna had run herself through the 23andMe DNA test. Having signed up through the 23andMe website, Anna received a testing kit within one to two days, which included a specimen bottle for a saliva sample and instructions on how to fill it. She returned the specimen to 23andMe in a pre-paid envelope along with a signed form. Three to four weeks later, Anna received an email indicating that her genetic data were available. She was then able to log into her account and access both her raw data and a basic report. The raw data is a huge file containing gene and SNP codes for approximately 1,500 genes and is not useful in any practical manner. However, I am able to process the file using my *GeneRx.ca* program to produce a report that is both informative and practical in terms of providing a diet, lifestyle and supplement protocol. Anna sent me her raw data file, and prior to our meeting I ran it through the program. Part of the report based on Anna's genetic profile (details at the end of this chapter) indicated the following:

- Significantly increased weight gain and hunger when consuming more than 22 grams of saturated fat per day
- Moderate increase in desire for energy-rich foods and increased weight gain with a low-protein, high-saturated-fat diet
- Higher risk of progressive weight gain and worse with a high-saturated-fat diet
- Overall, she handles carbohydrates well
- Increased inflammation with endurance exercise

By ignoring her genetics and following the latest "ketogenic" dietary trend, Anna not only failed to lose weight but actually gained more. In addition, the diet had caused an imbalance in the systems in her body and brain controlling feelings of hunger. The diet had also resulted in higher levels of inflammation, resulting in feelings of soreness, "puffiness" and fatigue.

Because of Anna's genetic coding, dropping her carbohydrates and increasing her calories from saturated fat led to increased fat accumulation, particularly around the abdomen, which posed a significant health risk. It also led to higher levels of her hunger hormone (ghrelin), which resulted in poor satiety and cravings for energy-dense foods. Restricting her carbohydrates was unnecessary as she actually coded well for these, and by doing so she limited her energy supply, leading to additional fatigue. Increased fatty weight contributed to increased inflammation.

Based on her genetics, I recommended the following protocol:
- Reduce her daily lean protein intake calculated according to her body weight
- Slightly increase whole grains to 2/3 the physical size of her protein portion
- Vegetables and salads allowed in unlimited quantities
- Reduce her saturated fat intake to less than 22 grams per day
- Supplements (see Appendix 2 for explanation)
    - Resveratrol Extra
    - Tri-Metabolic Control (TMC)

Anna lost three pounds in the first week and 16 more over the next eight weeks. The "puffiness" and inflammatory feeling were significantly reduced by day 10 and completely gone by two weeks. Energy levels, both day-to-day and with exercise, were back to normal by four weeks. At her two-year followup, Anna continued with a moderate and balanced diet and had maintained a healthy weight.

This is a good example of why there is no one diet that suits everyone. Diet trends come and go, and they work for some people but not others. In some cases, like Anna's, they can be detrimental. Genetics provides insight into your individual metabolism and allows a highly personal, safe and effective program to be designed.

Anna's Detailed Genetic SNP Coding

- APOA2: CC – significantly increased weight gain and hunger when consuming more than 22 grams of saturated fat per day
- FTO: TA – moderate increase in desire for energy-rich foods and increased weight gain with a low-protein, high-saturated-fat diet
- PPARG: GG – higher risk of progressive weight gain and worse with a high-saturated-fat diet
- TCF7L2: CC – handles carbohydrates well
- IRS1: TT – handles carbohydrates well

Note: Although I look at 59 genes and, through my GeneRx.ca *program, produce a 65-page report on my patients, for simplicity only the genes included in this book are used in these case reports.*

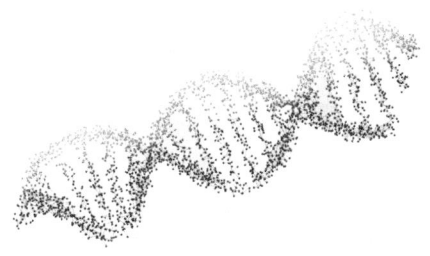

CHAPTER 3
DNA, Genes and SNPs (Single Nucleotide Polymorphisms)
A Brief History of DNA and the Science Behind SNPs

This chapter contains some detailed and interesting information relating to the field of DNA analysis. However, reading or understanding it all is certainly not essential for getting the most out of the remainder of the book. For those wishing to take a look at the important highlights, please skip to the summary section at the end of the chapter.

The concept of heredity is likely as old as the human race. The simple observation of inheritable traits such as eye and hair colour being passed from parents to offspring produced the earliest theories of character transfer. The philosopher Epicurus called these transferred essences "sperm atoms" even though half came from the mother. In Ayurvedic Medicine dating from the third and fourth centuries in India, a child's character is determined by four factors: the mother, the father, the mother's diet during pregnancy and the child's new soul. Not only does this recognize the influence of both parents, its recognition of the role of external factors was far ahead of Western thought. *The Ayurveda* was also perhaps the earliest text to hint at epigenetics (the ability to manipulate genes), recognizing the concept without any knowledge of the modern science that provides the background to this book!

In the late 19th century, Austrian scientist and friar Gregor Mendel performed a number of hybridization experiments on pea plants that helped establish the laws of inheritance, although his work was not truly recognized until 50 years later. Until Mendel, biologists had embraced the idea of "blending inheritance" by which parental traits were averaged into their offspring. Even Charles Darwin's weak "pangenesis" theory relied on the commingling of "gemmules." Mendel's work, rediscovered by Hugo de Vries and Carl Correns in the early 20th century, established "genotypic" inheritance, the modern understanding that characteristics are determined by genetic material and it is that material that is transferred from parent to child.

The existence of chromosomes, the cellular structures in cells that hold the DNA, had been known since the discovery of the microscope but their role as "vectors of heredity" was not established until late in the 19th century. With the rediscovery of Mendel's work in the early 1900s, German biologist Theodor Boveri and American physician Walter Sutton were able to relate the behaviour of chromosomes to the laws of inheritance, thereby laying the foundation for the determination of genetic material. Genes, the inheritable material conferring certain traits, were recognized as existing at specific locations on the chromosomes, and in 1913 Thomas Hunt Morgan's laboratory at Columbia University performed the first gene sequencing on the fruit fly, *Drosophila melanogaster*. Known as the "fruit fly scientist," Morgan and his team worked in the famous "fly room" at Columbia and provided many of the ground-breaking discoveries concerning the chromosomal theory of inheritance. He was awarded the Nobel Prize in Physiology in 1933.

The next piece of the puzzle was the determination that chromosomes and their genes had a complex molecule as their building block. That building block was DNA. Knowledge of this molecule had existed since the 1860s when Swiss chemist Johann Friedrich Miescher isolated "nuclein" from white blood cells, identifying it as having properties different from other proteins. Nobel Prize winner Albrecht Kossel in Germany isolated "nuclein" and gave it the modern name, deoxyribonucleic acid or DNA and documented the five chemical components that formed its "language": adenine (A), cytosine (C), guanine (G), thymine (T) and uracil (U).

Despite increasing evidence to the contrary, most scientists refused to believe such a simple molecule was responsible for all the information that created an organism. Protein molecules were still the front-runners as the potential chemical encoder of genetic traits. DNA simply didn't appear to have the variation in structure that would account for such tremendous diversity. This thinking started to change with the classic experiment of Frederick Griffith in the U.K.'s Ministry of Health pathology laboratory in 1928. It went like this:

The bacterium causing pneumonia exists in two types. A smooth surface (S) form that is highly virulent and a rough form (R), which is relatively benign. When injected into rats, the S-form is lethal whereas the R-form is not. Rats injected with S-form bacteria killed by heat survived. However, if the heat-killed S-form bacteria were mixed with live R-form bacteria and then injected, the mice died. What's more, blood from the dead rats contained *living* S-form bacteria! Something in the solution of killed S-form bacteria was "transforming" the R-form bacteria into the S-form and making them lethal.

What that "something" was remained elusive until 1944 when Canadians Oswald Avery and Colin MacLeod with American Maclyn McCarty at the Rockefeller University Hospital in New York isolated the "transforming principle" as DNA. Yet, despite their work, skepticism remained that this simple molecule was truly genetic material.

It was not until the Hershey-Chase experiment of 1952 (Hershey and Chase, 1952) that DNA was finally recognized without doubt as the genetic information of all organisms. These researchers studied viruses that attack bacteria (bacteriophages or "phages"). These organisms attach to the surface of bacteria and inject material that causes the bacterium to start producing multiple copies of the phage. This material, therefore, contained the genetic information of the phage and was known to be either protein or DNA. By tagging the protein and DNA separately with radioactive labels, they found that the infected bacteria contained phage DNA in their cells and not protein, proving finally that it was DNA that contained the genetic information of the phage organism.

Having established that DNA was indeed the molecule of inheritance, the challenge was to discover how its relatively simple structure could encode for something as complex as an entire organism from bacteria to humans. The discovery of the DNA double helix by Watson and Crick in 1953 is well known but their work was founded on the experiments of Chargaff and Franklin. Erwin Chargaff, an Austrian-Hungarian biochemist that left Germany in 1935 to work at Columbia University, proposed two rules based on his research. First, he noted that the number of guanine (G) units equalled the number of cytosine (C) units and the number of adenine (A) units equalled those of thymine (T). Second, he found that the percentages of the four units (G, C, A and T) were constant *within* a species but varied between species.

In 1950, Rosalind Franklin, a British biochemist from Cambridge University, joined the medical biophysics unit at the King's College Medical Research Council laboratory in London, England. Working with Raymond Gosling under the supervision of director John Randall, she used her expertise in X-ray diffraction to analyze purified DNA crystals. In this technique, called X-ray crystallography, X-rays are fired at purified molecules and their pattern of scatter is interpreted to define the molecular structure. It was slow and laborious work but by 1952 they had established the double-helical nature of DNA. The infamous "Photo51," taken by Gosling in that year, was critical in elucidating the structure but was not widely released as Franklin was leaving King's College. Wishing her work to stay in London, she gave a copy of the image to Maurice Wilkins, a New Zealand molecular biologist who had been working with her and Gosling. It was Wilkins that showed this photograph to Crick, visiting King's College in early 1953, paving the way for Watson and Crick's final revelation on the double-helical structure of DNA. There remains controversy over the circumstances of this transfer of information, which inevitably resulted in Franklin being largely and inappropriately forgotten in the history of DNA. Sadly, she died before Watson, Crick and Wilkins were awarded the Nobel Prize for Medicine in 1962, and as posthumous awards are not allowed, she remains largely unrecognized.

Francis Crick, a 35-year-old graduate student, and James Watson, only 23, were working together at the Cavendish laboratory of Cambridge University. They were focused on how complex genetic information might be encoded in a simple molecule. Using X-ray diffraction techniques similar to Franklin's, they began to theorize a structure for DNA that would explain its ability to hold such information *and follow Chargaff's rules*. Rosalind Franklin had provided further vital chemical interpretation when she advised Watson and Crick that their initial structural theories were impossible. The base pairs had to be at the centre of the molecule (being hydrophobic, that is, averse to interaction with water) while the nucleotide "backbones" had to be external (being hydrophilic or able to interact with water). Once Watson and Crick realized that base pairs A-T and C-G were of a similar size and structure and that the pairs were held by hydrogen bonds, formulation of the double helix structure was a logical step. This model also explained how, by uncoupling the two strands, the molecule could be replicated.

On March 19, 1953, Crick wrote a letter to his son, Michael. It began:

"Dear Michael, Jim Watson and I have probably made a most important discovery. We have built a model for the structure of des-oxy-ribose-nucleic-acid (read it carefully) called D.N.A. for short. You may remember that the genes of the chromosomes – which carry the hereditary factors – are made up of protein and D.N.A. Our structure is very beautiful."

This letter, sent just days before the formal announcement of his discovery, was sold at auction by Christie's in New York for $6.1 million in 2013, setting a new record for the sale of such an artifact.

On April 25, 1953, Watson and Crick published their "Molecular Structure of Nucleic Acids" in the journal *Nature* (Watson and Crick, 1953). It began in a most polite and unassuming manner:

"We wish to suggest a structure for the salt of deoxyribose nucleic acid (D.N.A.). This structure has novel features which are of considerable biological interest."

It concluded with a note of gratitude to the work of Wilkins and Franklin, and it was to change the face of molecular genetics forever. Its profound importance did not escape media attention with articles in London and New York appearing over the next couple of months announcing the discovery of the "secret of life."

In the coming years, Watson and Crick continued their work in Cambridge. Having postulated that the base sequence in DNA was responsible for carrying genetic information, they began to elucidate how this information was converted into the building blocks of cellular structure, proteins. Work by George Gamow, a Russian physicist who had defected to America and was better known for his work on the "big bang theory" in cosmology, established the link between DNA base-pair combinations and the 20 amino acids that were essential in the formation of all cellular protein. On the basis of this theory, Crick postulated that there was a messenger molecule that transferred the genetic information from the nucleus of the cell, which housed the DNA, to the cytoplasm, where proteins were manufactured. This molecule turned out to be RNA (ribose nucleic acid), similar to DNA but comprising a single strand and replacing the thymine base with uracil (U). The question remained, however, as to which base pairs coded for which amino acids.

The so-called "genetic code" was initially broken in 1961 by biochemist Marshall Nirenberg working with Heinrich Matthaei at the National Institutes of Health (NIH) in Maryland. Using a synthetic molecule of RNA and radioactively labelled amino acids, they established the first three-base code for a single amino acid: UUU coded for phenylalanine.

The next few years saw Nirenberg and his team at NIH in what has been called a "coding race" with Severo Ochoa, a Spanish biochemist working out of New York University Medical School. Between them they established the majority of "codons" (the base triplet codes for single amino acids).

Gamow had previously calculated that there were 64 possible permutations of the four base pairs, thus 64 codons. It turns out that some amino acids were encoded by more than one codon such that 61 codons code for 20 amino acids. Other codons act as "punctuation marks," breaking up the long sentences of base pair codons into "words" capable of producing a protein sequence. These include "start" and "stop" codons, also termed "nonsense codons" as they do not code for an amino acid. There are three "stop" codons, the first of which was discovered by Richard Epstein and Charles Steinberg and named "Amber" for the English translation of their friend Harris Bernstein (bernstein is German for amber). The theme was maintained as further stop codons were discovered and allocated "Opal" and "Ochre." There is only one principal "start codon," sadly hueless, and simply referred to by the base sequence AUG.

So, by the mid 1960s, DNA had been confirmed as the genetic material that allowed replication of cells and the transfer of inherited traits. The DNA, comprising organized sequences of base pairs coding for different proteins, was now known to be packaged into the cell nucleus in the form of chromatin, which is normally quite an amorphous mass of stretched-out chains. During cell division, this chromatin organizes into the neat, tightly packed and well-defined structures we know as chromosomes. The next big step was to begin the process of DNA sequencing, determining the order of nucleotides along the chromosome. This would give a complete picture of the organism's "genome" or total genetic makeup.

The first significant step in genome sequencing began in the early 1970s. Work was slow as early sequencing techniques were laborious, but by 1977, Frederick Sanger (known for determining the amino acid sequence of insulin), working at Cambridge University, had used DNA-polymerase and radiolabelled nucleotide bases to produce the first completely sequenced DNA genome, that of the bacteriophage (bacterial virus) phiX174. He also established a faster technique for sequencing called the "Sanger method" for which he was awarded the Nobel Prize in Chemistry in 1980. He used this method to analyze the first human DNA, the 16,569 base pairs of mitochondrial DNA and the same technique was eventually used to sequence the complete human genome.

Sequencing of simple viral genomes progressed rapidly, but it was not until 1995 that the Institute for Genomic Research, founded by American biochemist John Craig Venter in Rockville, Maryland, published the first complete genome (1,830,137 base pairs) of an independent organism, the bacterium *Haemophilus influenzae*. His use of a technique called "shotgun sequencing" proved to be a far faster way of analyzing DNA and he began to apply it to the human genome despite the belief that it was not as accurate as other methods especially for DNA of this size (3.3 billion base pairs).

At the same time as Venter, the Human Genome Project was underway. Originally proposed in 1985, it finally got underway under the auspices of the NIH in 1990 with a three-billion-dollar budget and an estimated 15-year completion. The project involved extensive international co-operation with teams in the U.K., France, Japan, Germany and China. Using a "hierarchical shotgun sequencing" method (also called "clone-by-clone"), researchers had sequenced about 80% of the human genome by 2001.

Venter's research, a private endeavour through his company Celera Genomics, contrasted ethically with the public project. Celera had announced a desire to establish patents on genes, preventing public access even for scientific research. The announcement by President Clinton in March 2000 that genome sequences could not be patented sent the biotechnology sector into a financial free fall, losing $50 billion in two days. In order to avoid potential problems, the public project released its initial draft sequence in July 2000, allowing unrestricted access. February 2001 saw the publication of articles in *Science* (Venter) and *Nature* (the international consortium) revealing details of the genome analysis along with insights into evolution and the value of the information to treat disease. The Human Genome Project was declared "complete" in April 2003, two years ahead of schedule, coincidentally coinciding with the 50th anniversary of the discovery of DNA. The project's surprising findings included the realization that there were only about 21,000 genes as opposed to the expected 100,000 and that only a third of genes appear to be involved in protein coding, previously believed to be the most crucial element in determining the characteristics of an organism.

As of 2018 the entire human genome remains about 99% sequenced with about 500 "gaps" that are proving remarkably difficult to analyze. How important these missing details are remains to be seen. The data is freely available in online databases including GenBank with other online resources adding additional information and analytical programs.

Research is currently focused on genetic variations between individuals called haplotypes. Besides referring to the set of genes inherited from one parent, haplotype also describes a cluster of inheritable single nucleotide polymorphisms (SNPs), which are variations at single positions in the DNA sequence among individuals. As the DNA sequence of any two individuals is 99.9% identical, the 0.1% variation coded within these haplotypes is almost entirely responsible for differences in everything from hair and eye colour to metabolism and disease risk. The International HapMap project was founded in 2002 to document these variations but was decommissioned in 2016 as a result of cybersecurity issues. It has since been superseded by the 1000 Genomes project (1KGP), which was initiated in 2008 and completed in 2015, having reconstructed the genomes of 2,504 individuals from 26 populations. It was published in the journal *Nature* in October 2015 and reported a resource of over 99% of single nucleotide polymorphisms. This has provided the foundation for the interpretation of human genetic analysis and therapeutic intervention such as epigenetics and nutrigenomics that are the subject of this book.

From DNA to Protein – How Genes Become Working Molecules

The genes discussed in this book code for proteins that play a vital role in the absorption, metabolism and storage of energy sources. They may act directly by influencing a process such as transportation of a nutrient. The gene FABP2, for example, codes for a protein that plays a vital role in the transport of long-chain fatty acids across the gut wall. A variation in the coding for this gene (associated with the rs1799883 SNP A-allele) results in the protein having twice the affinity for these fatty acids, a property that has a profound influence on fat absorption and storage. Genes may also act indirectly by coding for proteins that influence hunger and satiety mechanisms designed to control food intake. The FTO gene, for example, codes for the enzyme alpha-ketoglutarate-dependent dioxygenase. The A-allele of the rs9939609 SNP in this gene is associated with higher levels of the hunger hormone, ghrelin, and resistance to the satiety hormone, leptin.

To understand how a SNP can influence a protein, it is important to clarify the basic mechanism by which a DNA sequence, a gene, becomes a protein such as an enzyme or a cellular receptor. This process is called transcription.

Most people are aware of the terms DNA, gene and chromosome. Some clarification is required as, to a certain extent, they are all part of the same organization of genetic material.

- DNA is the double helix containing the "genetic code"
- One DNA strand may be up to five centimetres in length but is folded tightly within the cell to form a chromosome. These chromosomes become visible during cell division when they "condense' and organize into the structures we commonly recognize as chromosome shapes

- Each cell (except sperm and egg) has two copies of each chromosome (DNA strand), one from each parent
- Genes are certain sequences within a strand of DNA. One DNA strand may have up to 1,300 genes and be up to 250 million base pairs in length
- Genes vary in length from around 27,000 to two million base pairs

We have seen how a DNA molecule comprises a double-stranded helix made of nucleotide base pairs, each base pair forming a rung of the spiralling ladder. The outer "hand-rails" are made of phosphate and sugar molecules. A gene is a section of this ladder and can be anywhere from 27,000 to two million "rungs."

The nucleotides in DNA provide the "alphabet," the letters of a language that codes for the protein expressed by a certain gene. There are four of them: adenine, thymine, guanine and cytosine. Along one strand of the DNA molecule, they can occur in almost any order, but on one rung, attached to the complementary strand, adenine is always paired with thymine, and guanine with cytosine. This is a vital structural necessity for the process of DNA replication. The coding sequence for a gene therefore comprises a sequence of nucleotide bases on one strand of the DNA molecule.

Proteins comprise a chain of amino acids and are therefore structurally similar to DNA. As we saw above, the way in which DNA codes for a protein sequence is analogous to a language. If the DNA nucleotide bases are the letters, then each three-base sequence on one strand can be considered a word. These words are termed "codons." There are 64 possible permutations of the four base pairs, thus 64 codons. As it turns out, some amino acids are encoded by more than one codon such that 61 codons code for the 20 amino acids. Other codons act as "punctuation marks," breaking up the long sentences of three-base codon words into meaningful sentences capable of producing a protein sequence. These include "start" and "stop" codons, also termed "nonsense codons" as they do not code for an amino acid.

The process by which a gene sequence becomes a functional protein involves processes that include both the translation of the code and its editing. The process is complex and involves a number of steps. One of the reasons for this is that the gene contains many sequences that do not actually code for any of the amino acids in the protein. These sections of the DNA strand are called "introns." The sections that actually provide code for the protein are called "exons." For example, insulin, well known to be responsible for controlling glucose levels and, overall, one of the most important metabolic proteins, is a chain of 21 amino acids. The gene responsible for coding this protein (INS on chromosome 11) has 1,430 base pairs, enough information to code for 470 amino acids. Therefore 95% of the DNA is non-coding intron. Getting the meaningful insulin "sentence" out of this DNA "chapter" is where the translational complexity occurs.

From gene to protein:
1. The DNA double helix splits into two separate strands through the middle of each "rung." This process occurs within the cell nucleus and is instigated by the enzyme RNA polymerase. This enzyme is directed to start splitting the DNA at the start of the gene sequence by means of a promoter region, a sequence of non-coding DNA (or intron) at the beginning of the first coding section (exon) of the gene.
2. Once split, the bases that make up each rung are exposed, one on each side. The RNA polymerase enzyme then uses one of the strands as a template to form a molecule called messenger RNA (mRNA), which is the molecule that will eventually provide the information to make the protein. Only one side of the DNA helix, the "coding strand," holds the code to the protein. The other strand is used to make the mRNA and is called the "template strand." mRNA is like a single strand of DNA with the same nucleotide bases (except for thymine being replaced by uracil). By pairing bases with the template strand, the mRNA therefore resembles the coding strand in its sequence of bases. The process of forming the mRNA molecule is called **transcription**.
3. The mRNA molecule created from the template strand is an exact copy of the coding strand of the DNA and therefore

contains both coding (exon) and non-coding (intron) sequences. In order for it to code only for the amino acid sequence of the protein, it needs to be edited and have the non-coding sequences removed. This process is called "splicing."
4. The initial RNA strand is actually called pre-mRNA. With splicing it becomes the mRNA that is able to code for the protein. The splicing process, as with transcription, occurs in the cell nucleus.
5. The spliced mRNA can now move out of the nucleus into the cytoplasm of the cell, the manufacturing area. Here it binds to "factories" called ribosomes, where the information on the mRNA is used to build the protein. Having identified the "start" sequence, each three-base code leads to the addition of the appropriate amino acid, creating a chain of them or polypeptide. Once created, this polypeptide undergoes structural modification to form the final active protein. The process of forming a protein from the mRNA is called **translation**.

DNA Strand Terminology

The DNA molecule consists of two strands joined through the nucleotide bases that form the rungs of the helical ladder. One of these strands holds the code for the protein manufactured by each gene. This is called the "coding strand." It also called the mRNA-like strand, the sense strand or the positive (+) strand. The other strand is used as a template to make the mRNA that is eventually translated into the protein molecule. This is the "template strand," also called the anti-sense strand or negative (-) strand.

By convention, it is the coding (+) strand that is sequenced in DNA analysis, and most commercially available platforms (including 23andMe) use this protocol. However, a few platforms use the template (-) strand, and this can lead to confusion when interpreting SNP alleles. For example, if a platform using the coding (+) strand reports a variant SNP as "A," then one using the template strand (-) will report it as "T."

Relevance to SNPs

By understanding the above mechanism, the impact of a single change in a base pair such as a SNP becomes apparent. A different base within a DNA exon will result in a similar change in the mRNA and an altered three-base code for one position. This will most often lead to a different amino acid being substituted, possibly having a profound effect on the structure and function of the protein produced. Changes in the non-coding intron might lead to alterations in the start or stop points or affect splicing, again leading to changes in the structure, quality or quantity of the protein.

SNPs and Mutations

We have seen that in the human genome of three billion base pairs, individuals differ by only 0.1%. Thus, 99.9% of the entire genetic code is identical. That 0.1% accounts for the differences between us. The explosion in the speed, accuracy and availability of modern genetic analysis has answered some questions but posed many more as our understanding of the complexities of genetic coding and transcriptional control grows. The Human Genome Project, the first foray into whole-genome sequencing, had a budget of three billion dollars and a time frame of over 10 years. Current techniques have reduced the cost to $3,000 and it can be performed in 24 to 48 hours. However, while this has allowed tremendous advances in genetic medical research and fuelled an entire industry based upon personalized genomics, definitions and terminology have become blurred. This is partly the result of technology outpacing language and understanding in the field and partly the result of popular commerciality offering a simplified and easily comprehensible vocabulary to the consumer. Negotiating this new genomic jargon is important if one is to avoid misinterpretation and inappropriate context.

What is a SNP (Single Nucleotide Polymorphism)?

The vast majority of personal genetic analysis involves the detection of SNPs (pronounced "snips"). A SNP is a difference in a single nucleotide of one base pair in a DNA sequence. For example, at a specific point (locus) in a gene, the population might show two different sequences:

TGG**C**AG and TGG**T**AG

In this case, there would be a SNP at position four. (In reality, of course, gene sequences are far longer, and a SNP may occur at position 12 or 972, for example.)

SNPs are extremely common and occur approximately once every 1,000 nucleotides, resulting in approximately four to five million of them in an individual's genome. They most often occur in the non-coding control regions between genes and therefore have the potential to exert a profound effect on gene expression. Some occur in the coding or exon region and have an effect on the final protein product. Thus far it appears that the vast majority of them have no discernible effect on health, disease or phenotype (the appearance or function of the body). However, a small (but increasing) number do appear to have an impact on metabolism, immunity, inflammation, neuroendocrine function and detoxification. SNPs can be highly individual or shared across large populations, thus providing clues to ancestry.

> **How Does Ancestry Testing Work?**
> 1. *SNP analysis: compares your SNP profile to databases of previous tests. Variability arises as different companies have different databases and some ethnic groups may be less well represented, resulting in biases in database content. This is the most useful testing from a genealogical perspective.*
> 2. *Y-chromosome analysis: as the Y chromosome is passed on exclusively from father to son, this test is useful for the male ancestry line and is often used to evaluate whether two families with the same surname are related. It is not as helpful for genealogy as it only looks at one family line.*
> 3. *Mitochondrial DNA: DNA exists not only in the nucleus but also in small organelles in the cell cytoplasm called mitochondria. These are the "power houses" of the cell and responsible for producing energy to run the organism. Mitochondrial DNA is passed from the mother to both male and female offspring and therefore can be used to examine the female ancestral line. Again, as it only looks at single families, it is not very useful in determining ethnic origin.*

From our perspective, we are interested in SNPs that affect disease risk, physiologic functioning such as metabolism, response to supplements or pharmaceuticals, and susceptibility to environmental toxins or stress. For most complex diseases such as diabetes or heart disease, risk is determined by multiple SNPs, and it is the interaction between these that provided the most important insight into personal health.

Mutations

The original term "mutation" was used to describe any rare change in the DNA nucleotide sequence that is usually associated with disease. This change can be inherited from the parental sperm and egg DNA and is termed a germ line mutation. Changes that occur during the lifetime of an individual, either spontaneously or, for example, from exposure to radiation, are called somatic mutations. There are a number of major classes of DNA mutation. Some of these involve the sequence of the DNA itself, whereas others involve insertion or deletion of DNA segments. For example:

1. Point mutations: These involve a change in one DNA base pair with the substitution of one base residue for another. This may result in a change in one amino acid in the protein the gene codes for (missense mutation) or a failure to build the protein at all (nonsense mutation). **This is clearly analogous to a SNP, the distinction being the frequency with which point mutations occur and the seriousness of their consequence.**
2. Insertions or deletions: These may involve one or two base pairs or whole sections of a gene or chromosome. The resulting disruption of gene function can be substantial. For example, deletion of three nucleotides at position 508 in the gene coding for cystic fibrosis trans-membrane conductance regulator leads to a loss of the amino acid phenylalanine at position 508 in the protein product. A small error, but it causes cystic fibrosis, a severe and life-threatening disorder of the lungs and intestinal tract. Insertions or deletions can also result in a

"frameshift mutation" where transcription is shifted due to a deleted or inserted base pair.
3. Chromosome gain or loss: Normally there are two copies of each chromosome. Adding or losing an entire chromosome can have a profound effect. For example, having three copies of chromosome 21 results in Down's Syndrome.
4. Translocation: Translocation of part of a chromosome involves no loss of genetic material but the transfer of one part of a chromosome to another. For example, transfer of a part of chromosome 9 to chromosome 22 gives rise to the "Philadelphia Chromosome" associated with chronic myeloid leukemia.

Interestingly one of the most common "mutations" in human DNA is the G-T mismatch. It occurs once in every 10,000 to 100,000 base pairs. Normally G would only pair with C, and T with A, but it appears that base pair mismatches not only occur but remain unrecognized by the cell's DNA repair mechanisms. Somehow the two bases alter their chemistry so they "fit" and avoid disrupting the DNA. Why this happens, whether other mismatches occur and the role this has in disease are other avenues for exploration in this ever-expanding field.

SNP versus Point Mutation

A common question that arises is the difference between a SNP and a point mutation. After all, they both represent alterations in the DNA code, affect gene function and are heritable. Both can be passed on to offspring. Until recently SNPs were defined as single point mutations that occurred in 1% or more of the general population. This arbitrary number was a consensus formed before the advent of NexGen multiple parallel gene sequencing. At that time, assembling multiple individual genomes formed the reference genomic baseline template against which a single DNA genome could be compared. Differences that were considered "rare" were defined as mutations, while those that were common (greater than 1%) were considered "polymorphisms." The majority of these common polymorphisms involved just a single base-pair change and were called single nucleotide polymorphisms or SNPs. It was also believed that mutations caused disease whereas polymorphisms did not.

As NexGen sequencing has progressed and multiple complete individual genomes become sequenced across a population, the line between "common" and "rare" has become blurred. Differences considered "mutations" in some population groups are found to be present in over 1% of other groups and are therefore considered "pleomorphisms" and vice versa. In addition, many of these rare mutations that were thought to be disease-causing remain harmless or even beneficial in some groups. For example, sickle-cell anemia is caused by a SNP (SNP rs334) and results in an abnormality in the beta chain of the hemoglobin protein in red blood cells. While the disease is rare (less than 1%) in developed nations, populations in countries where malaria is endemic have prevalence rates estimated at 10 to 40%. The reason is that the sickle-cell trait confers protection against malaria without causing sickle cell disease, a condition that is frequently fatal for infants in these countries. This "genetic advantage" results in the mutation being passed down through generations rather than being eliminated by natural selection. This is just one example, and as population genomes are explored, there appear to be many more.

The other blurring between SNPs and point mutations occurs with respect to disease. Research increasingly demonstrates that certain SNP alleles are associated with illness such as diabetes or cancer. SNP abnormalities in the promoter region affect methylation while exon SNP mutations directly affect protein structure. An example is the BRCA1 SNP, a tumour suppressor gene implicated in the development of breast cancer. Although rare in the general population (1 in 400), its prevalence in the Ashkenazi Jewish community is 2.5%. Thus, although technically a SNP as it has a specific population prevalence greater than 1%, it imparts serious disease risk. The definitions of "mutation" and "pleomorphism" therefore need further clarification before using them in the wider field of personal genomics and personalized therapies. An example is individualized cancer treatment where therapies target individual mutations within the cancer cell.

However, if this "mutation" is actually a polymorphism and present in all somatic cells of an individual, then treatment would be toxic to all cells. A second example demonstrates how two subsequent mutations are required to produce disease risk. A population may have a heritable or "germline" SNP that predisposes them to disease risk, but it is only when a secondary somatic (acquired) SNP occurs that the disease becomes manifest. For example, meningioma risk is increased with the germline SNP SMARCB1, but tumours occur only when a somatic mutation in the *NF2* gene is superimposed.

A recent study (Jones, 2015) looked at how genome analysis of cancer cells alone could potentially affect treatment. The researchers then repeated the process, sequencing both the cancer cells *and* the individual's germ line DNA. They found that many mutations or pleomorphisms considered mutational in the cancer cells were actually "normal" for that individual and present in all their cells. This obviously would have a profound effect on treatment. Such information is vital in an era of increasingly personal genomic-based medicine.

SNP Terminology

The standard terminology for defining a SNP includes three details:
1. The name of the gene, usually relating to the protein product it codes for. For example, FABP-2 or Fatty Acid Binding Protein 2.
2. A reference code. For FABP-2, this is Ala54Thr. It refers to the position on the gene at which the SNP occurs and, in this case as it is a SNP occurring in an exon, the amino acid substitution that is coded for. The normal or ancestral coding results in an alanine residue at position 54 of the FABP-2 protein, while the variant coding leads to a threonine residue.
3. An "rs" number, which is the SNP registration number. For FABP-2, this is rs1799883.

There may also be a chromosome "position" number, which refers to the location of the SNP on the chromosome relative to a genome assembly point. (For FABP-2, this is chromosome 4 119320747). This information, however, is more of interest to researchers.

An "allele" is a variant form of a gene SNP. Humans have two copies of each gene and the combination of the two is termed the "genotype." (The copy on one chromosome is called a "haplotype.") If an individual has the same gene allele on each chromosome, they are termed "homozygous." If the two genes have different alleles, they are termed "heterozygous." Some gene alleles are dominant or recessive depending on how they influence the appearance or function of the body (phenotype). Dominant alleles "overpower" recessive alleles to exert their effect. Thus, the phenotype coded by the gene will be present in those that are homozygous for the dominant gene or heterozygous (one dominant and one recessive). Only those homozygous for the recessive allele will fail to show the trait or express the recessive allele trait.

For example, there are two alleles of the hairline gene. The allele for a straight hairline is recessive while the allele for a V-shaped hairline is dominant. If we call the recessive allele "S" and the dominant allele "V," then individuals with the genotype VV or VS (or SV) will have a V-shaped hairline and only those with SS will have a straight hairline.

Some diseases are caused by recessive alleles, such as sickle cell disease. Those related to genes not on the X or Y sex chromosomes are called "autosomal" while those on the X or Y chromosomes are called "sex-linked" or "X- or Y-linked." X-linked traits are more common and include diseases such as colour blindness, hemophilia A and B, and Duchenne muscular dystrophy.

However, most traits and diseases are polygenic, that is, influenced by a number of genes. Eye colour is an example and explains why we can have green and hazel eyes, caused by a mixture of blue and brown alleles even though the blue allele is recessive.

When performing SNP analysis and describing variants, we will be comparing one individual's coding to a "baseline" or "standard" allele.

This baseline allele is also called the "ancestral allele" (and sometimes the "wild allele") and refers to the original evolutionary haplotype. Subsequent mutations that occurred during human evolution have produced "derived alleles" and represent the SNP variation between individuals that we use to analyze personal traits.

> **Allele Synonyms**
>
> **Normal allele**: *ancestral allele, standard allele, wild allele, reference allele.*
>
> **Variant allele**: *risk allele, derived allele, mutant allele, atypical allele.*

The ancestral allele is typically determined by genetic analysis of a species close to us on the evolutionary tree, such as the chimpanzee or Macaque monkey. Although used as a reference, it is typically not identified in most SNP analyses. It can be found in databases such as the dbSNP Data Dictionary (https://www.ncbi.nlm.nih.gov/snp). The ancestral allele can be the most frequent allele in the human population but not always. In some cases, the ancestral allele has been largely replaced by a derived allele, indicating active evolution. The gene ALDH5A1 codes for an enzyme that breaks down the neurotransmitter GABA. It is important for cognition and has been associated with overall cognitive ability and the preservation of mental function in the elderly. Population studies have shown that a derived allele of this gene is replacing the ancestral gene, likely as a result of the conferred survival advantage the allele imparts. However, in most cases it would seem that derived alleles are less advantageous and are more highly associated with disease than are ancestral alleles. The reason for their existence and survival despite causing a phenotypic disadvantage is a subject of much conjecture and likely relates to our human ability to modulate evolutionary pressures.

For a given SNP, the alleles will be defined according to the amino acid base variation and are often labelled as ancestral or baseline (the "normal" or original allele) and derived or variant (the "mutated" allele). Alleles may also be labelled "major" or "minor" according to their population frequency. The minor allele is most often (*but not always*) the derived or variant allele and may also be the "risk" allele as it usually (*but again, not always*) confers an adverse health effect. The prevalence of this allele in the general population is sometimes listed along with the other information for the SNP and is termed the MAF (minor allele frequency).

SNP Allele Terminology

For example, if the ancestral allele is C, then the original or baseline "normal" coding for a particular gene might include the following sequence:

*...GTG**C**AT, where "C" is the SNP*

As there are two copies (one on each chromosome) of the gene, there would be two SNPs and these would both be ancestral, thus CC.

If the variant (derived or risk allele) is T, then the gene sequence would read:

*...GTG**T**AT...*

The individual may only have this on one of their two chromosomes and have the ancestral allele on the other. Their coding would therefore be CT (the ancestral or normal allele usually goes first), and they would be termed heterozygous. If both genes have the variant, then they would be TT and termed homozygous.

Another value often assigned to a SNP allele includes the Risk Ratio, a measure of the degree to which the allele imparts advantageous or deleterious health effects, supported by research references.

The Risk Ratio (or Relative Risk) is a value that defines the ratio of the likelihood of an event occurring in a test or exposed group versus the likelihood of the event occurring in a control or non-exposed group. For example, if the risk of developing lung cancer in smokers (exposed group) is 17% and the risk in non-smokers (non-exposed or control group) is 1%, then the Relative Risk of developing lung cancer in smokers is 17 divided by 1, which equals 17. Smokers are 17 times more likely to develop lung cancer.

Colour coding is often used in reports to allow rapid interpretation of an individual's SNP genotype. Green is applied to the genotype that is homozygous for the normal, major or ancestral allele, yellow for the heterozygous state and red for those homozygous for the variant, minor (usually the "risk") allele.

An individual will have a genotype defined by the two alleles that make up the SNP. For example, for FABP-2, the normal allele is G and the variant allele is A. The genotype will be listed as GG, GA or AA, and each will have its own health implications as follows:

GG = homozygous normal
GA = heterozygous (note that the normal allele is always listed first for heterozygotes)
AA = homozygous variant

> ### SNP Nomenclature and Orientation
>
> *The nomenclature for certain SNPs can be confusing in the literature. Although the rs number remains the same, the allele description can be inconsistent. Most of the time this relates to whether the coding (+) strand or the template (-) strand is referenced (see DNA Strands above). As nucleotides are in pairs (A-T and G-C), what may be an A-allele on one strand is automatically a T-allele on the other. This is also termed "strand orientation."*
>
> *For example, the NR3C2 gene codes for the mineralocorticoid receptor and has the SNP rs5522. The standard format indicates alanine (A) is replaced by guanine (G) at position 538, such that codon 180 changes from ATT to GTT. This leads to replacement of an isoleucine (I) with a valine (V) in the final protein (technical terms NRI180V or NR3C2 c.538A>G). This would make A the normal or reference allele and G the risk or variant allele. Most research papers studying the NR3C2 SNP use this terminology, as does SNPedia. Some sources, including 23andMe refer to the inverse strand and "flip" the bases such that A (normal) becomes T and G (risk) becomes C.*
>
> *Anomalies such as these occur from time to time, and mostly relate to changes in the reference DNA database used and the DNA strand reported.*

Personal Genetic Testing

Current personal genetic testing incorporates two components. One is the genetic analysis, which is the actual genotype analysis and identification of your individual SNP alleles. The second is the decoding process, which assesses SNP genotypes and produces a statement of disease risk or lifestyle impact.

Genotype analysis is now accessible to everyone with companies providing "direct to consumer" marketing. They provide "raw data" usually in the form of a huge text file that lists many thousands of genes and SNPs. This file is generally not helpful to an individual as it only includes information such as the SNP rs number, your coding and possibly the normal and variant alleles. To get any useful information about your health risks, you need to have that data decoded. Some companies provide their own decoding or may suggest a third-party site where you can upload the data in order to get a usable report. Costs vary from $200 to $3,000 depending on how much of your genome gets sequenced and how much data is interpreted. They may offer lifestyle, diet or supplement suggestions to mitigate potential risks identified in your analysis. SNP selection in these decoders is important, as the vast majority of SNPs have no known impact on health. Sorting out the clinically relevant SNPs from those that do not currently appear to affect disease, lifestyle or physiologic function is also important. Genetic testing may give a list of 20 SNPs for a certain gene yet only two are relevant in terms of health or disease.

The FDA has given approval for the testing of certain conditions in which certain SNPs significantly increase risk. These include Parkinson's disease, macular degeneration, late-onset Alzheimer's and celiac disease along with rare conditions such as Factor XI deficiency blood clotting disorder and MUTYH-associated polyposis, which has an increased risk of colon cancer. However, they have cautioned against some tests or reports that predict patient response to certain medications, arguing that the clinical evidence is not supportive and that the information may be used inappropriately by patients or physicians to discontinue medications that are necessary. Such caution is advisable in the context of "what can help can harm" and underlines how interpretation of genetic data and the use of such information need to be carefully monitored, particularly when the consequences are profound. The NIH-based National Human Genome Research Institute is currently working to improve regulation of genetic testing to maximize accuracy and consistency in the areas of analytical validity, clinical validity and clinical utility. These last two relate to the value of assessing and treating risks associated with SNPs and ensuring they lead to improved health outcomes.

What Is Genotyping versus Sequencing?

Genotyping is a DNA analysis technique that looks at the specific variants an individual has in their DNA. It looks for the existence of known genetic polymorphisms by examining localized areas of someone's DNA rather than analyzing the entire DNA sequence. The variants searched for comprise the "chip" or microarray and may be a small number focused on a particular aspect of health, such as exercise, or an extensive selection providing a more comprehensive picture. This technique is efficient, cost-effective and accurate and is used by most major commercial platforms such as 23andMe. The value of this technique lies in its ability to reveal variations that have known influence and, in terms of the genes we are looking at, can most often be influenced by treatment interventions.

DNA sequencing (Next Generation sequencing, or NGS) determines the exact sequence of the DNA strand including areas that are constant between individuals and the areas where variants occur. By not looking for specific variants, this technique can identify polymorphisms that are unique to an individual. Although the entire human genome can be sequenced using NGS, this is time consuming and still very expensive. In addition, it provides a huge amount of information that would not be considered useful for our purpose. Companies therefore analyze areas considered important, notably the regions coding for proteins (exons), leading to the term "Exome" analysis. While providing much of the same information as genotyping, sequencing offers a large amount of data that may not be understood, such as variations that, thus far, do not have any known influence on health and are not amenable to treatment. Sequencing can also look for methylation tags.

If we consider your DNA as a book, then genotyping looks for altered letters in specific words, while sequencing reads the entire sentence and looks at every word for any difference. While more comprehensive and providing a better overview of the "story," sequencing reveals a lot of words whose meaning is unknown. Genotyping on the other hand looks at specific words that have known meaning and therefore offer the potential for "editing" (treating).

What is important to understand in the context of the above discussion is that having a risk allele for a condition does not mean you have or will develop that condition. For diseases such as cancer or Alzheimer's, there is tremendous potential for tests to induce anxiety, which in itself provides a health risk. Discussion with a health provider familiar with genetic testing before *and* after the test is tremendously important in terms of defining expectations, allaying fears and planning sensible and effective intervention.

Of the available platforms, I have encountered a number of issues that make them difficult or unhelpful when it comes to using your genetic data to make useful lifestyle improvements.

Our aim is to provide practical and usable information with comprehensive and easy-to-follow treatment options that make sense according to your genetic data.

Chapter 3 Summary

What is DNA?
DNA is the material in every cell of your body that provides the blueprint to manufacture essential functional components called proteins. Proteins include important molecules like insulin, antibodies and muscle. Proteins affect and control all the processes in your body including how you handle food in your diet, your metabolism, when you feel hungry and where you store energy.

What is a gene?
A gene is simply a section of the long DNA strand that includes the information for one particular protein. Each DNA strand has many genes along its length. Your genes are inherited from your parents so there are two copies of each one: one from your mother and one from your father.

How does the gene make a protein?
The DNA information of a gene forms a code. The code comprises a sequence of letters, forming "words" in a sentence that the machinery in the cell can "read" to get the instructions to make the protein. A change in the gene code letters of a word will affect the sentence, possibly making it unintelligible or possibly altering its meaning and ultimately affecting the final protein product.

What is personal genetic testing?
Companies that analyze your DNA run a test that searches for "spelling mistakes" in certain "words" in your gene "sentences." These mistakes or variations are called SNPs, pronounced "snips."

What is a SNP ("snip")?
A SNP is a variation in the letters that make up the code of a certain gene.

For example, say a gene contains the word TA**G**ACT as part of its coding sentence. Certain individuals in a population might have a "spelling mistake" or variation in this word, which makes it read TA**C**ACT. The SNP is at the third letter and can be a G or a C. The two words may make the entire gene sentence read differently such that the final protein product is altered. That alteration can affect an important function such as how you respond to sugar.

What does my "coding" mean?
Your DNA analysis looks at many different genes that are known to have certain common spelling mistakes or SNPs. These SNPs are associated with different conditions and traits, including everything from hair and eye colour to heart attack risk. SNP coding refers to the letters that are different in a SNP.

Using the example above, you might code G or C for that gene. The G and C are called "alleles." As you have two copies of each gene, you have two alleles so you could be GG, GC or CC.

Research studies have ascertained that some alleles are associated with an increased risk of certain conditions such as diabetes or cardiovascular disease. They may also affect things such as your ability to handle carbohydrates in your diet, your ideal fat intake or your tendency to gain or lose weight. By referencing results from your DNA test, this book will give you information about diet, health, metabolism and weight based on your gene coding.

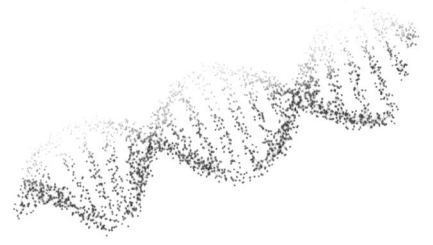

CHAPTER 4

SNPs, Disease and Epigenetics

Understanding SNP Terminology and Relevance: The Influence of Diet and Lifestyle on Gene Expression

This chapter contains some detailed and interesting information relating to SNPs, their effects and how they can be modified. However, reading or understanding it all is certainly not essential for getting the most out of the remainder of the book. For those wishing to take a look at the important highlights, please skip to the summary section at the end of the chapter.

Now that we understand what a SNP is, it is important to start looking at how they affect our physiology and health and why they increase our risk of disease. We can then use that knowledge and our genetic coding data to institute a highly personalized treatment plan.

As we have seen, there are four to five million SNPs in the human genome, and it is currently thought that the vast majority have no effect whatsoever on cellular function, human phenotype or disease risk. However, the number of SNPs that do appear to influence human function and illness is growing year by year. The SNP resource *SNPedia* currently has over 100,000 SNPs with that number doubling roughly every 12 months. Information is based on research examining SNP allele variance across populations and associating it with prevalence of disease.

So how do we know that particular genes and their SNPs are associated with certain diseases or health risks? This information comes from a number of sources, the most important of which are genome-wide association studies (GWAS).

Genome-wide association studies are used to identify genes that are involved in the development or progression of human disease. Such studies have been tremendously important in SNP analysis and provide a novel way to analyze the factors that contribute to complex illnesses such as obesity, diabetes and heart disease. They are also very valuable at interpreting the influence of factors such as diet, stress and the environment on the expression and impact of these genetic variations.

The completion of the Human Genome Project and the International HapMap Project has created a massive database of reference human genes. This database lists genes for which common variations (SNPs) occur along with their frequency. By comparing these variations to a "germ line" or "ancestral" database (usually chimpanzee DNA), the original coding and the variants that occur in the human population can be determined.

In a GWAS, the DNA of thousands of individuals with a disease is compared to that of a similar population without the disease. The frequency with which a certain SNP coding occurs in each population will identify whether or not that coding is associated with the disease. Determining association is, of course, different from assigning causality, although in many cases the molecular biology behind the association has been determined or alluded to. The rapidity with which the process can be completed for multiple SNPs across large populations has led to a vast body of research being produced covering diseases as diverse as age-related macular degeneration (AMD; leading to blindness), type 2 diabetes and Parkinson's disease.

As the National Human Genome Research Institute states in a *Genome-Wide Association Fact Sheet (2015)*:

"The impact on medical care from genome-wide association studies could potentially be substantial. Such research is laying the groundwork for the era of personalized medicine, in which the current one size-fits-all approach to medical care will give way to more customized strategies. In the future, after improvements are made in the cost and efficiency of genome-wide scans and other innovative technologies, health professionals will be able to use such tools to provide patients with individualized information about their risks of developing certain diseases. The information will enable health professionals to tailor prevention programs to each person's unique genetic makeup. In addition, if a patient does become ill, the information can be used to select the treatments most likely to be effective and least likely to cause adverse reactions in that particular patient."

One of the earliest GWAS looked at risk factors for heart attack (myocardial infarction). Researchers looked at 92,788 gene-based SNPs in patients that had sustained a cardiac event and compared them to matched controls free of heart disease (Ozaki, 2006). They found that certain SNPs were significantly more prevalent in the heart attack group, most notably those associated with the gene coding for lymphotoxin-alpha (LTA). One SNP, in particular, had an Odds Ratio of 1.78 when individuals were homozygous for the at-risk coding. (An Odds Ratio above 1 signifies significantly increased risk.)

In another landmark GWAS, researchers looked at a SNP in the context of age-related macular degeneration (AMD). Analysis of 116,204 SNPs yielded a significant association with the complement factor H gene (CFH). Individuals homozygous for the risk allele had an Odds Ratio of 7.4 for developing AMD (Klein, 2005).

> **Relative Risk (also called Risk Ratio) and Odds Ratio**
>
> **Relative Risk** is a value that defines the ratio of the likelihood of an event occurring in a test or exposed group versus the likelihood of the event occurring in a control or non-exposed group. For example, if the risk of developing lung cancer in smokers (exposed group) is 17% and the risk in non-smokers (non-exposed or control group) is 1%, then the Relative Risk of developing lung cancer in smokers is 17 divided by 1, which equals 17. Smokers are 17 times more likely to develop lung cancer.
>
> The **Odds Ratio** is a statistical value that quantifies whether one event is likely to lead to another, that is, how closely associated two events are. For example, using the lung cancer figures, if 17% or 17 out of 100 individuals exposed to smoking develop lung cancer, then the odds of developing the disease in smokers is 17 divided by 83 (number that smoked but didn't get cancer), which equals 0.205. Only 1 in 100 non-smokers develop cancer so the odds in this group is 0.01. The Odds Ratio is the first figure divided by the second, 0.205/0.01, which equals 20.5. If this figure were 1, then it could be said that smoking does not affect lung cancer. If the number is greater than 1, then smoking leads to a higher risk of cancer. The greater this number is, the higher the risk. And 20 is very high.

Of course, an association with a disease is not necessarily a *cause*, and in some cases the functional effect of the SNP cannot be clearly related to the abnormal physiology or pathologic process. However, in many cases it can be explained either by inference from knowledge about how the gene functions or directly through laboratory research. For example, taking LTA (lymphotoxin-alpha) SNP and the risk of heart attack, the variant risk allele causes a twofold increase in cell-adhesion molecules in coronary arteries, considered a potential cause of blockage and spasm. In AMD, the risk variant leads to complement molecule deposition in the small vessels of the eye with subsequent plasma leakage. Zinc supplementation slows the progression of AMD as it has been shown experimentally to control CFH (Complement Factor-H) gene function.

Certain genes have well-documented and researched function, which the variant SNP alleles are shown to affect. This might be through a change in the final translated protein product. For example, the intestinal fatty-acid binding protein-2 gene (FABP-2) plays a very important role in the absorption and binding of both saturated and unsaturated long-chain fatty acids from the GI (gastro-intestinal) tract, also called the digestive tract. The gene contains the SNP Ala54Thr (rs1799883), which affects sensitivity to saturated fats and refined carbohydrates. The variant allele (A) increases production of the gene product (fatty-acid binding protein-2) such that even moderate amounts of fat or carbohydrate in the diet result in weight gain, glucose and insulin resistance, and an unhealthy lipid profile including lower levels of the "good" high-density lipoproteins (HDL) and higher levels of the "bad" low-density lipoproteins (LDL) and cholesterol. Thus, the three genotypes produce these effects:

AA = Significantly increased sensitivity with a twofold increase in fatty acid uptake
GA = Moderately increased sensitivity
GG = No appreciable increased risk

Another example is the gene APOE (coding for apolipoprotein-E), which makes a protein that combines with fat to form a very-low-density lipoprotein called apo-lipoprotein-E. It removes cholesterol from the blood stream and therefore has a beneficial effect on heart disease risk. This gene is also associated with the development of Alzheimer's disease. The gene contains two SNPs in its exon (protein-coding region) with normal and variant alleles at each one. An individual inherits one APOE gene from each parent. This results in four different potential alleles, called E1, E2, E3 and E4. (In practicality, the E1 allele does not exist so there are only three alleles in the general population.) E3 is the most common allele and considered the "baseline." The three alleles produce lipoprotein products of the same name—APOE2, APOE3 and APOE4, differing by one amino acid base. This subtle change results in a significant alteration in an individual's risk of developing Alzheimer's. Those with the E2-allele have a lower risk than baseline, while those with the E4-allele have an increased risk 11 times normal. If you have two E4-alleles your risk goes up to 25 times the normal risk.

However, it is important to realize that, unlike hemophilia for example, having the risk allele does not automatically mean you will get the disease. It is perfectly possible to have two E4-alleles and never develop Alzheimer's. Part of this relates to the multifactorial nature of the disease and the involvement of numerous genes. This is where interpretation becomes more difficult, and the interacting role of other gene SNPs needs to be taken into consideration. For example, for the APOE gene, the role of the APOA2 gene needs to be factored in. The APOA2 gene affects the absorption of ingested fat from the GI tract. The presence of a variant allele of this gene that increases fat absorption when combined with the APOE E4-allele would make the likelihood of Alzheimer's disease far more likely.

Another way that a SNP may affect gene function is if it affects the regulatory region and therefore the *quantity* of the gene product rather than the *quality*. The variant C-allele of the MC4R gene (rs17782313) is linked to the production of fewer MC4 receptors. This results in impaired satiety feedback within the hypothalamus of the brain and subsequent increased food intake leading to higher body mass index (BMI).

> **Body Mass Index (BMI)**
>
> BMI is a basic measure of obesity determined by dividing your body weight in kilograms by the square of your height in metres.
>
> For example, if your weight is 65 kilograms and your height is 1.67 metres, then your BMI = $65/1.67^2$ = 23 (kg/m^2).
>
> As a measure of health:
> BMI < 18.5   Underweight
> BMI = 18.5 to 24.9   Normal weight
> BMI = 25 to 29.9   Overweight
> BMI > 30   Obese

The examples above are relatively straightforward and involve a one-to-one association. In this regard, they are similar to disease-causing "mutations" such as sickle-cell anemia in which an abnormality in the hemoglobin molecule in red blood cells causes distortion and damage, which is caused by replacement of the amino acid glutamine with valine at the sixth position of the beta-chain. However, many of the diseases we will be considering are multifactorial, diseases such as type 2 diabetes, metabolic syndrome and obesity. There are multiple genes and subsequently multiple SNPs associated with these conditions, and the body of research concerning them is extensive and growing. I have chosen SNPs based on their relevance, the body of evidence to support their associations and their ability to be manipulated by interventions such as diet, lifestyle, exercise and natural supplementation.

An example of such a SNP would be the FTO (Fat Mass and Obesity Gene) SNP rs9939609. In large-scale multiple population GWAS, the risk allele (A) accounts for an overall 1% increase in BMI and a 22% increased risk of obesity, *independent* of diet and exercise. However, the effect is significantly worse if an FTO-A individual consumes a low-protein, high-saturated fat or high-calorie diet. Adults with the variant risk allele (A) tend to consume, on average, 125 to 280 more calories per day than T-allele carriers. The overall effect of the A-allele is quite profound with heterozygote (TA) carriers weighing an average 1.2 kilograms (2.6 pounds) more than TT individuals. Homozygote (AA) carriers weigh an average 3 kilograms (6.6 pounds) more than TT individuals and have a 1.67-fold higher rate of obesity than TT, rising to 2.5 times if ingesting a high-carbohydrate or high-fat diet. This trend is seen as early as age seven and continues throughout life. The variant allele is also associated with an increased risk of developing type 2 diabetes and metabolic syndrome. Fortunately, the influence of the gene can be counteracted by dietary changes and increased exercise. Adopting a low-fat, low-sugar, higher protein diet, minimizing saturated fat and exercising regularly are recommendations for those carrying this allele.

Treating Our Genetics

The above example touches on how we can effectively intervene in order to maximize our metabolic efficiency and minimize risk imparted by our genetic SNP coding. There are a number of approaches we can use for intervention.

Nutrigenomics
Nutrigenomics is the science that studies the association between genes, diet and health. Emerging over the past 10 years following completion of the Human Genome Project and HapMap/100 Genomes projects, it aims to replace the use of simple general physiology with a more personalized assessment of the interaction between genotype and nutrition. In terms or "personalized nutrition," nutrigenomics can propose the optimal diet for a certain genotype. In terms of "personal health," it can recommend a diet that minimizes risks imparted by an individual's genotype.

As an example, the MC4R gene SNP rs17782313 is associated with increased BMI. Each variant (C) allele results in an 8% increase in obesity risk and increases BMI by 0.22 units. It is associated with insulin resistance and a 14% increase in risk of type 2 diabetes. Those homozygous for the variant allele (CC) show up to a 43% increase in body weight. Using a low-calorie diet with restricted saturated fat and simple sugars along with intermittent fasting (I.F.) helps control weight and may reduce the risk of developing diabetes.

Another good example is the rs5082 SNP of the APOA2 gene. The variant C-allele is associated with reduced APOA2 transcription and a markedly increased BMI and obesity risk when consuming a high-saturated-fat diet. For an individual carrying the C-allele, diets high in saturated fat (such as ketogenic diets) will have a highly detrimental effect and promote weight gain. Keeping saturated fat below 22 grams per day is shown to completely mitigate the effects of this variant SNP allele.

Gene Modulation
Just because you have a certain gene coding does not necessarily mean it has to exert its effect. Many of the metabolic genes only appear to be "active" under certain circumstances. By avoiding those circumstances, the adverse effect of the gene is not realized. Its action is effectively "turned off."

An example would be the FTO SNP rs9939609. The risk allele (A) is associated with a slightly increased risk of obesity independent of diet and exercise. However, if an individual consumes a low-protein, high-fat, high-carbohydrate diet, then its effect is significant. It leads to an increase in hunger, particularly for energy-dense foods, reduced satiety, excessive food consumption and increased weight gain. Adults with the variant risk allele (A) tend to consume, on average, 125 to 280 more calories per day than T-allele carriers. The overall effect of the A-allele is quite profound. Compared to individuals with TT coding, AA carriers weigh an average 3 kilograms (6.6 pounds) more and have 2.5 times the risk of obesity when ingesting a high-carbohydrate or high-fat diet. If an AA individual adopts a higher protein, low-fat, low-carbohydrate diet, they can effectively "turn off" this gene, restoring their hunger-satiety balance to normal and controlling their weight.

Nutrigenomics Examples
- **APOA2**: The association between the variant allele of the APOA2 gene, high BMI and a high-fat diet is one of the strongest examples of such interactions. A mean increase in BMI of 6.2% is seen in CC versus CT or TT individuals when consuming equally high amounts of saturated fat exceeding 22 grams per day. This association is of particular importance in societies with abundant food and a diet high in fat content (such as a typical western diet). Compared to CT and TT, individuals with the CC genotype have been shown in multiple populations to be at a significantly increased risk of obesity when they ingest more than 22 grams of saturated fat per day. The risk is substantial with an average 6.2% increase in BMI. However, the difference does not appear to exist when fat intake is below this threshold.
- **PPARG**: The G-allele predisposes to a low BMI. So having the G-allele would appear to be highly beneficial. However, in an environment where food is readily available and fats are a significant part of our diet, the G-allele may end up being detrimental. While the G-allele provides an initial protection against obesity and diabetes, a persistently poor diet will eventually lead to increased adiposity, and this seems to reverse the effects of the allele. In fact, once BMI increases, the risk of further weight gain and the development of diabetes go up. Once an individual becomes diabetic, then the G-allele confers an increased risk of diabetic complications.
- **FABP2**: A-allele carriers (homozygous AA or heterozygous AG) are far more likely to have increased serum glucose levels both after fasting and after a large meal rich in saturated fats and sugars. In addition, the amount of saturated fat consumed appears to have a profound effect on how much the A-allele affects each individual.

> The North American Pima Indian population living in Arizona has one of the highest prevalence rates of obesity and type 2 diabetes in the world. However, a genetically identical population, with a similar high incidence of the A-FABP2 allele, living in rural Mexico demonstrates no such tendency (Schulz 2015). The difference in metabolism can be traced to the change in diet and activity level resulting from the Arizona population assuming a "North American" lifestyle incorporating poor diet and low levels of exercise. A study in the journal Metabolism (Chamberlain, 2009) found that people with genotypes AA or AG that ate a diet containing 53 grams or more of saturated fat per day had lower HDL to total cholesterol ratios; higher cholesterol, LDLs and triglycerides; and higher insulin resistance (as seen by higher levels of HOMA-IR, a biomarker of insulin resistance). The recommendation was for limited saturated fat intake in A-allele carriers.
>
> - **TCF7L2**: A study from 2012 (Phillips, 2012) found that female T-allele carriers had increased risk of metabolic syndrome (Odds Ratio = 1.66), elevated insulin levels and insulin resistance, increased BMI and adiposity, and higher blood pressure than did CC homozygotes. The study also found there to be a strong epigenetic dietary component. High-saturated-fat intake increased the Odds Ratio of metabolic syndrome from 1.66 to 2.35 and was associated with further impairment of insulin sensitivity.

Epigenetics

Epigenetics is the field of study that looks at how biologic mechanisms can turn genes on and off. As opposed to the "gene modulation" example above, the mechanisms in epigenetics actually stop the expression of a gene, that is, they prevent it from producing a protein. Thus, alterations in the phenotype of a cell or an individual can be achieved without changing the genetic code. And unlike the "gene modulation" example, epigenetic changes are heritable, passed on from cell to cell or from parent to offspring.

Consider the maturation of stem cells into differentiated cells. This happens all the time during embryonic development. All cells have the same DNA, but genes are selectively turned on or off to effect changes in how the cell appears or performs. The process by which this occurs is called **DNA methylation**. Adjacent to most genes is a *promoter site* through which the gene can be turned on or off. These sites contain **"CpG islands,"** repeating C-G sequences. Methylation occurs at the cytosine base. When it is converted to 5-methylcytosine (5mC) by methyltransferase enzymes (DNMT), it leads to a diagonal molecular arrangement that alters function, as diagrammed below:

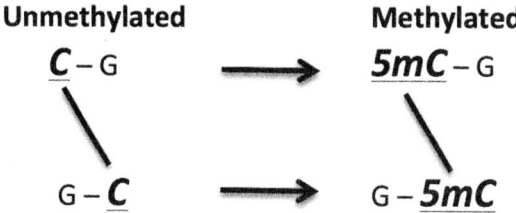

While about 80% of CG sites are methylated, the vast majority of CpG islands in normal tissues are unmethylated. General hypermethylation can be associated with cancer as it leads to silencing of tumour-suppressing genes. Focal hypomethylation has also been shown to increase cancer risk by allowing activation of genes and increasing the impact of DNA mutation. Methylation in intergenic areas reduces the risk that mutations will lead to altered gene expression.

Methylation in a promoter sequence effectively prevents transcription and "silences" the gene. Removal of the methyl groups turns it back on. Methylation can be transient, and there is evidence that in some genes this occurs on a daily basis according to circadian rhythm. Other sites can remain methylated for years and be passed on as cells divide. Females have two X-chromosomes, one of which is effectively silenced for life through methylation and histone modification (a structural change, which compacts the DNA into a untranscribable form called heterochromatin).

Significant alterations in DNA methylation can have a profound impact. Patients with hereditary sensory/autonomic neuropathy have an autosomal dominant mutation, which causes abnormal function in one of the DNA methyltransferase enzymes (DNMT1) that is essential to adult neural maintenance. Although the condition only reduces overall methylation by about 8%, its specific impact on the brain results in early neurodegeneration and dementia. Similarly, Fragile X Syndrome, a condition associated with developmental delay and cognitive impairment, is caused by hypermethylation and subsequent silencing of a gene responsible for a protein essential for protein synthesis at synapses.

Methylation is one of the three principal epigenetic mechanisms listed below that are known to control gene expression.

> ### Mechanisms of Epigenetic Gene Silencing
>
> - *DNA methylation*
> - *Histone modification*
> - *Non-coding RNA-associated gene silencing*

It was originally thought that such modification of gene expression could not happen once a cell had matured. However, that assumption has proven to be remarkably incorrect. Research over the past 10 to 15 years has demonstrated how environmental and personal factors can impart epigenetic changes that lead to inheritable adverse health effects.

As all cells contain the same DNA information, it is the *expression* of certain genes that makes cells different in the body—a nerve cell versus a skin cell, for example. We might term this "Nature." It controls development and function within an individual. It makes us different from someone else in terms of everything from hair and skin colour to temperament and emotional stability. However, many genes can be controlled by external factors such as environment, diet, stress and exercise. We might term this "Nurture." Both nature and nurture can affect our health and predisposition to disease. It also appears that at least some "nurture-induced" epigenetic changes can be inherited.

There are numerous examples of how the environment can impact health through epigenetic mechanisms. Children born during times of famine have less methylation of the IGF2 gene and develop an increased risk of heart disease and obesity (Painter, 2005; Heijmans, 2008). Others have been shown to have an increased risk of schizophrenia (Clair, 2005). Air pollution has a dose-dependent effect on histone acetylation in rats (Dinga, 2016). It increases acetylation, which leads to increased transcription, a possible cause of increased lung disease. Youth growing up in a lower socioeconomic status have increased DNA methylation tags on genes related to depression (Swartz, 2017). The serotonin transport gene SL6A4 encodes a protein essential for the transport and activity of serotonin, a neurochemical known to have low activity in depression. Increased methylation of the gene reduces transcription and therefore serotonin activity. Individuals with increased methylation of this gene had more response within their amygdala (the brain area responsible for interpretation and emotional response to threat) and a higher incidence of post-exposure depression.

Mice with a specific neurological disorder (similar to Kabuki syndrome in humans) are unable to grow new cells in a part of the brain associated with learning. This is due to a defect in the enzyme histone deacetylase (HDAC). HDAC de-acetylates DNA, allowing the tightly folded chromatin structure into which it is normally packed to open up and permit transcription. These mice demonstrate low activity in this enzyme and subsequently reduced transcriptional ability, which affects cellular development. The condition can be reversed with the addition of beta-hydroxybutyrate (BHB), a chemical with the ability to open up chromatin in a similar way to HDAC. Giving mice BHB or feeding them a low-carbohydrate ketogenic diet (which naturally increases BHB levels) results in a reversal of the learning deficiencies in these mice and increased cell proliferation within the brain (Shimazu, 2013; Bjornsson, 2015).

> **Environmental Factors Affecting Methylation**
>
> - Particulate air pollution (PM)
> - Bisphenol-A
> - Cadmium
> - Chromium
> - Lead
> - Mercury
> - Polycyclic Aromatic Hydrocarbons (PAHs)
> - Persistent Organic Pollutants (POPs) such as pesticides, solvents and plastics
> - Tobacco smoke

The DNA methylation pattern in human newborns is affected by maternal exposure to toxins. A Mexican study (Rojas, 2015) looked at the effects that maternal exposure to low levels of arsenic exposure in drinking water had on DNA methylation patterns in offspring. They found significant alterations in DNA methylation in cord blood cells, particularly in genes related to growth and development. There was substantial correlation with gestational age, birth weight, placenta weight and head circumference. Other heavy metals including chromium, mercury, lead, cadmium and selenium have been implicated as causing changes in DNA methylation, affecting a number of genes including those involved in transcriptional regulation and apoptosis. It is postulated this may play a role in carcinogenesis.

Particulate and chemical air pollution including nitrous oxide, sulphur and polycyclic aromatic hydrocarbons (PAHs) have a profound effect on the health of those living in cities. One European study (De Prins,

2013) found a substantial correlation between exposure to these pollutants and decreased global methylation levels. Other studies have found associations between air pollution and the methylation of genes involved in asthma morbidity in both children and the mothers of children with respiratory ailments (Sofer, 2013). Pre-natal exposure to particulate air pollution (PM) causes hypomethylation of the leptin gene, a possible link to leptin resistance and increased BMI in children raised in industrial environments (Saeden, 2017). PAH and PM are linked to hypomethylation in genes associated with oxidative stress, inflammation, DNA repair and cell-cycle regulation, suggesting a potential mechanism for such adverse health effects as asthma, cancer and dementia.

> ### The Future of Gene Editing
>
> *If it were possible to edit gene methylation, then we could potentially turn genes on and off without actually affecting the DNA or genetic code. Researcher Liu used CRISPR technology to guide enzymes involved in the methylation/demethylation process to specific gene loci (Liu, 2016). When applied to a specific promoter gene important in the growth and development of new neurons (BDNF), demethylation caused the gene product to increase by two to three times. The researchers also found they could reprogram cells by turning certain genes on and off. They applied their methylation program to fibroblast cells and induced them to form muscle proteins, thereby indicating significant potential to alter gene expression and affect the fate or function of a cell. It could also provide potential treatments for DNA methylation-related disorders such as cancer, lupus and cardiovascular disease.*

Epigenetic Effects of Stress

Scientists at the Emory University School of Medicine in Atlanta took a group of male mice and conditioned them to associate the smell of acetophenone with electric shock (Dias, 2014). They subsequently became fearful of the smell alone, which would cause shuddering. The mice also developed more M71 receptors, the specific smell receptors that enabled them to detect the acetophenone at much lower levels. The researchers then took sperm from these mice and impregnated females. When the offspring were exposed to acetophenone they shuddered in a similar manner, even though they had never been exposed to the smell before. The same was true for the next generation of mice. When exposed to other smells, the mice did not shudder. The offspring had more M71 receptors in the brain than did controls and expressed the same epigenetic marker on the gene encoding for M71 as did the grandfather mice. They were also found to have global pattern changes in transcription within areas of the brain associated with stress responsiveness including increased expression of cortisol-activated genes.

The pervasiveness of chronic stress in our 21st century society is no longer a surprise to most people. Yet its very pervasiveness means we ignore it. Unfortunately, that may have a lasting effect on generations to come, not simply because the burden of treating many stress-related diseases will fall upon our younger population, but because it appears our chronic stress is changing our genes in a way that is detrimental to our children even if they do manage to remain stress-free.

In a study performed at New York's Mount Sinai Hospital (Yehuda, 2016), researchers analyzed the genes of Jewish men and women who were interned in concentration camps, witnessed or experienced torture, or had to hide during the Second World War, as well as the genes of their children. Compared to a control group that lived outside Europe during the war, they found that the children born to Holocaust survivors had significantly higher levels of anxiety and stress disorders. Epigenetic tags were found on genes associated with trauma and stress in both the Holocaust survivors and their offspring but were not found in the control group or their children.

The above are examples of epigenetic inheritance, whereby altered gene expression is inherited in the same way as genetic code. It has profound implications in terms of health. Factors such as stress, poor diet and exposure to toxins that have a detrimental effect on one generation can be passed on to the next. The accumulation of genetic dysfunction over multiple generations will inevitably lead to progressively deteriorating health and increased incidence of disease.

The precise impact of traumatic stress on DNA methylation and how that translates into increased risk of disease and poor mental health is currently under investigation. It is certainly true that early life stress, including pre-natal stress, results in lifelong abnormalities in metabolic, endocrine, immunological and neural function and is a major risk factor in psychiatric disease. There is good evidence that at least part of the effect is mediated by alterations in receptor status in the HPA (hypothalamic-pituitary-adrenal) axis. Traumatic stress has a profound effect on the methylation of exons coding for glucocorticoid receptors and serotonin transporters with hypermethylation leading to significant reduction in gene expression. These methylation patterns are heritable and are passed on to the offspring of adults with conditions such as post-traumatic stress disorder (PTSD).

A number of studies evaluating the children of adults that experienced trauma such as famine (Heijmans, 2008), the Holocaust (Yehuda, 2016) and the Montreal Ice Storm (Cao-Lei, 2014) provide evidence for the transmission of epigenetic traits. Additionally, there appears to be a predisposition to the development of certain trauma-related conditions including PTSD in terms of methylation patterns, particularly for genes involved in immune and nervous system function. What's more, it appears that these changes may be modified by treatment, as certain methylation markers were improved following therapy for PTSD.

There is good evidence for the association of methylation with anxiety and depression. In one study of identical twins, methylation patterns in the twin affected by early-onset major depression were substantially different from those of the unaffected sibling (Malki, 2016). Differences in methylation can occur from a number of sources with epigenetic influence being most important. In one study (Lester, 2018), children that received low levels of maternal care had increased stress responsiveness and hippocampal reactivity to cortisol with altered methylation of the glucocorticoid gene promoter. Although epigenetic, this might be considered a form of behavioural modification and not truly heritable.

Finally, the importance of stress in the expression of variant genotypes is not to be underestimated. In one study looking at the association of the variant MC4R C-allele with obesity, once adjusted for other variables, the results indicated that those individuals with high stress levels had a stronger association with higher BMI and preferential intake of processed and fat-dense foods over fruits and vegetables. The authors concluded that the interaction of stress and the variant allele of MC4R altered energy intake and eating behaviour to an extent that exceeded that of the variant allele alone (Park, 2016). Further discussion on this topic can be found in Chapter 17.

> ### *Methylation and Aging*
>
> *There is increasing evidence that levels of methylation across the genome influence aging and that a number of epigenetic factors can affect this process. Research has characterized genes that become either hypermethylated (over-methylated) or hypomethylated (under-methylated) compared to baseline. While there are genetically inherited methylation sites, the vast majority of the genome is programmed with "age zero" methylation, cells being essentially pluripotent.*
>
> *As we age, methylation patterns emerge and allow development and growth. The activity of methylation pathways obviously changes over time with the greatest activity occurring during embryogenesis and childhood. There is tremendous variation in these methylation levels across tissue types. Sperm and egg cells (gametes) remain "age zero" for life as does placental tissue. Female breast tissue ages more quickly than all other tissues and brain tissue more slowly. Interestingly, men age more quickly in methylation terms as do women that have later menopause. Brain function deteriorates as methylation age increases. While there*

is a general increase in DNA methylation as we age, certain sites demonstrate a trend toward reduced methylation. A theory that there is an epigenetic program running in all cells that turns genes on and off at various times in life provided the base for the "Epigenetic Clock" revelation of Steve Horvath (Horvath, 2013).

Steve Horvath grew up in Germany, and along with his twin brother and a friend formed a discussion group called the Gilgamesh Project (inspired by the Sumerian epic poem of the same name that was written in the second millennium BC and describes the King of Uruk's search for a plant that can restore youth). The three decided to dedicate their lives to prolonging healthy human life.

Steve Horvath, now a professor of Human Genetics at UCLA, analyzed available DNA methylation data to produce a "multi-tissue age-predictor" which correlated chronological age with methylated-DNA (DNAm). He looked at 353 DNA methylation sites. He found that methylation levels did not relate to cell age or number of divisions and was not directly related to levels of gene expression as might be expected from methylation's effect on transcription. DNAm represents what he calls "an epigenetic maintenance system" or "epigenetic clock" that ticks at a similar rate across many body tissues and varies in rate according to the age of the person not the cell. For example, a newly produced white blood cell from a 50-year-old will carry the DNAm signature of a 50 year old, not of a new cell. It is accurate in predicating age to within 1.5 years.

The clock is clearly important, as "methylation age" is a better predictor of disease and mortality risk than chronological age. It offers the potential for measuring the effects of anti-aging therapies and might one day allow treatment of age-related disease.

> *Interestingly, individuals with accelerated aging (progeria), subject of the movie* The Curious Case of Benjamin Button *or those with a rare condition that never age (Syndrome X), show normal DNAm aging. This would indicate that these conditions involve epigenetic factors besides DNAm or are a result of abnormal biochemistry beyond gene expression. Some individuals show accelerated DNAm aging independent of other factors. For example, individuals with a history of significant trauma, stress, PTSD and major depressive disorder (MDD) have a significantly higher rate of epigenetic aging, and this likely relates to their increased risk of disease development and early death. Chronic stress is associated with neurochemical and neuro-hormonal abnormalities as well as structural changes in the brain such as hippocampal shrinkage and poor amygdala-frontal integration. However, not all individuals have the same reaction to stressful trauma. Only an estimated 20% develop PTSD, for example.*

It is clear that whatever genetic cards we are dealt, we have the potential to modify their effects. We can work with them to maximize metabolic efficiency and prevent them exerting any adverse effects on our health. We can "turn on" the good genes and "turn off" the bad, combining diet, lifestyle and supplements. We can change our diet to the optimal balance as determined by our metabolic SNPs and incorporate exercise to further enhance energy balance. Lifestyle changes are also important to reduce the epigenetic influence of pollution and stress.

Chapter 4 Summary

What SNP information will I get from my DNA test?
For each gene you may receive the following:
- The name of the gene, for example, FTO.
- The "rs" number, which is a numeric reference code. For example, for FTO this is rs9939609.
- The "normal" allele, which is usually the most common in the population and the one typically imparting the lowest risk to your health. For example, for FTO the normal allele is T.
- The "risk" allele, which is usually the less common allele and the one typically imparting an increased risk to your health. For example, the risk allele for FTO is A.
- Your allele coding or genotype, which are the alleles you have as determined by your DNA analysis. For example, for FTO you may be TA.

Why are some SNP alleles called "risk"?
- Researchers carry out Genome Wide Association Studies (GWAS).
- A GWAS analysis looks at DNA data from a large population and whether a certain SNP allele is associated with a certain disease.
- If people with a certain allele are more likely to have the disease, then this allele is called a "risk" allele.

If I have the "risk" allele, will I definitely get the disease?
- No. For the genes we are discussing, there are numerous factors that influence whether or not you develop a condition. In addition, not everyone expresses their risk genes, meaning their effect is "turned off." This may occur as the result of other genes or by non-genetic influences such as diet.

Do all "risk" SNPs cause disease?
- No. The majority of the genes we are looking at affect your ability to handle certain food types (such as carbohydrates), your metabolism and your ability to lose or gain weight.
- Some have associations with metabolic diseases such as diabetes as a secondary effect.

What can I do if I have "risk" alleles?
- Just because you have a certain gene coding does not necessarily mean it has to exert its effect. Many of the metabolic genes only appear to be "active" under certain circumstances. By avoiding those circumstances, the adverse effect of the gene is not realized. Its action is effectively "turned off."

How do I "turn off" my risk alleles?
- By changing your diet to fit your genes. This is termed "nutrigenomics."
- Nutrigenomics is the science that studies the association between genes, diet and health.
- By changing your lifestyle to fit your genes. This is termed "epigenetics."
- Epigenetics looks at how personal and environmental factors can influence gene activity.
- These factors include stress and exercise.
- Supplements. Certain natural supplements can be beneficial

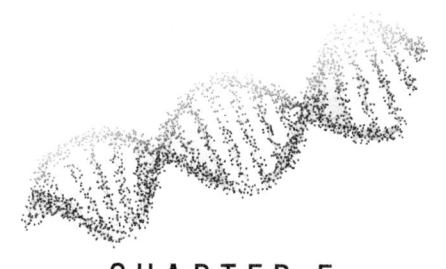

CHAPTER 5
Case Study #2
Diet, Weight and Diabetes

George is a 61-year-old construction worker. Although not significantly overweight, he had struggled over the years with periods of unwanted weight gain and subsequent dieting. His main concern when he came to see me was that his blood sugars and inflammatory markers were beginning to rise and his general practitioner (GP) had warned him that he was pre-diabetic.

For the past year, he had been trying to limit grains, starches and fruits to just one meal a day with moderate fats, higher protein and an abundance of vegetables and salads. When he was very diligent with his diet (lower calorie, carbohydrate and fat), he lost weight and his blood sugars improved. What he really struggled with was consistency, that is, sticking to the diet for any prolonged period of time. Any diet would result in him feeling hungry all the time. He would also begin to experience significant and hard-to-ignore food cravings, particularly for unhealthy, higher fat, energy-dense foods.

George's genetic profile included the following coding:

- FTO: AA – low metabolic rate, requires high protein
- PPARG: GG – good weight loss with calorie restriction
- ADIPOQ rs17366568: AA – low adiponectin during weight loss; needs low fat and carbohydrate

- ADIPOQ rs17300539: GG – lower adiponectin during weight maintenance
- TCF7L2: CT – increased glucose and insulin response to carbohydrates
- APOA2: TC – increased LDL, weight and inflammation with more than 28 grams of saturated fat

George's TCF7L2 coding makes him prone to type 2 diabetes, and this risk is increased by the low adiponectin resulting from his FTO and ADIPOQ genotypes. Although beneficial at present, his PPARG GG coding makes him susceptible to diabetic complications. His FTO and ADIPOQ coding also result in significant food cravings and a tendency to eat high-fat foods. He tolerates these poorly because of his PPARG and APOA2 coding with increased weight and inflammation.

Based on his genetics, I recommended the following protocol:

- Protein at 1.2 grams per kilogram of body weight per day (divided between meals)
- Intermittent fasting
  - Two meals per day with one small snack in between **only if needed**
  - All food to be consumed within an eight-hour period
  - 16 hours fasting
- Grains or starches at one meal per day but keeping the size to ½ the size of the protein and eliminating fruit and sweets for the first eight weeks. After eight weeks, he could eat them at two meals per day, keeping the portion size the same.
- Saturated fat to a maximum of 28 grams per day
- Calories 800 to 1,000 per day
- Tri-Metabolic Control – two capsules 30 minutes before lunch and dinner for eight weeks and then cycle it in one week out of every four weeks. This helped to boost his low adiponectin, lower ghrelin and regulate leptin to control food cravings, hunger and inflammation, as well as boost his metabolic rate.

- Metabolic Xtra – two capsules twice a day on an empty stomach to help stabilize his blood sugars while he gained control over his diet
- Start a regular aerobic exercise program (significant benefit with FTO AA)

Within one week, George's food cravings and hunger had been significantly reduced, and at the two-week mark he had little to no desire to cheat on his diet. By four weeks his blood work including his blood sugar had normalized. He lost the 10 pounds he had gained and his weight remained stable. Just over three years later, he has maintained his weight, his blood work remains normal with no pre-diabetic status and his cravings are under control.

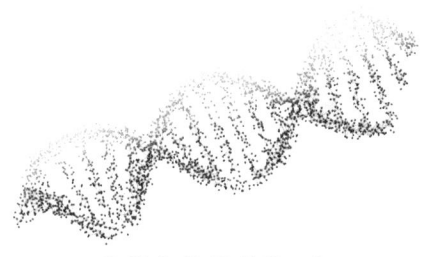

CHAPTER 6
Which Genes, Which SNPs?
How We Chose the Gene SNPs for This Book

When deciding which SNPs to cover in this book, we took into account a number of factors. After all, there are a vast number to choose from! As previously noted, any one individual will differ from a reference genome by about four to five million SNPs. Around 10,000 of these affect protein coding while 500,000 influence expression through changes to non-coding regions. The number associated with complex genetic phenotypes such as diabetes and obesity can be estimated by looking at available research from genome-wide association studies (GWAS). The NCBI (National Center for Biotechnology Information) provides a searchable database (ClinVar) of 62,000 genetic variations, which can be filtered according to type and association with disease.

A search for SNPs associated with diabetes produces over 5,385. However, narrowing the search to include only those with likely clinical influence reduces this number to 349. Doing the same for "obesity" yields 3,414 SNPs with 314 being likely pathogenic, which is a little more manageable but still not particularly practical. In order to incorporate SNP analysis into my practice, I have narrowed the numbers down using the following criteria:

1. **Availability**: Many of the SNPs are not analyzed by commercially available kits such as 23andMe. I currently only use SNPs that appear as part of the standard testing chips.

2. **Research**: The SNPs I use have significant research to support their involvement in disease. Research includes genome-wide association studies, basic science research, and *in vitro* (laboratory-based) and *in vivo* (organism-based) analysis and clinical data.
3. **Relevance**: I use SNPs that are relevant to common conditions and diseases that affect my patients.
4. **Treatability**: I choose SNPs that are amenable to treatment by changes in diet and lifestyle or through natural supplementation.
5. **Integrative**: I include SNPs that interact with others to influence their expression and degree of impact on health.

My *GeneRx.ca* platform looks at 59 gene SNPs covering a number of categories including metabolism; carbohydrate, fat and protein handling; exercise; stress response; immunity; inflammation; detoxification and neurotransmitters. Some SNPs will be included in more than one category, given their scope of influence.

The *GeneRx.ca* medical professional report is a 65-page, comprehensive, in-depth analysis covering multiple areas of health and fitness. It allows your health-care practitioner to provide you with a thorough profile of your strengths and weaknesses and to institute a treatment protocol that maximizes your health and reduces disease risk. (See additional information below.) Such a complex and individual approach is not practical for a book, and I have therefore elected to present gene SNPs that, in my opinion, have the widest impact in the majority of individuals. They are often the most important and the most commonly discussed, and they provide the greatest opportunity for effective intervention. They address issues that I see daily in my practice, such as diet, meal timing, weight, stress and inflammation.

Chapters on specific SNPs include a discussion of the gene and its role in health, diet and metabolism. Genotypes are explained in terms of the "normal' and "risk" alleles with information on how these affect you as an individual. Treatment suggestions are then offered and include recommendations for diet, exercise, lifestyle and supplements. I often advise an eight-week "Genetic Retraining" period during which time the treatments are more extensive or stringent. This period is important in that it helps break the cycle of poor nutrition and health that many of us find ourselves in. Once completed, a more relaxed maintenance regimen is instituted.

Eight-Week Genetic Retraining

On average, I find it takes about eight weeks of treatment to maximize the function of a gene or optimize its expression. This is why, for some gene SNPs, I suggest an initial eight-week program that incorporates more rigid dietary changes and enhanced supplementation. Following this period, you have the opportunity to "relax" a little, knowing that your genetically idealized metabolism can now cope with wider choices. That's not to say you can jump right back into old habits! Your genes remain sensitive to the fuel they are given, and a return to an unhealthy lifestyle will eventually undo all the retraining!

For the first eight weeks, it is important to follow all the dietary and supplemental suggestions as closely as possible. If you are allowed simple carbohydrates at one meal per day ½ the physical size of your protein, then do not start consuming those carbohydrates at two meals per day or ¾ the size of your protein after the first week. If you do, then the retraining process will take much longer or will not happen at all.

After eight weeks, once you have diligently retrained your genes, you now ease back a little and enjoy the benefits of your balanced hormones and genes. You must still keep your protein and saturated fat intake at the same level, as this is a key factor for health as determined by your genetic profile. What can vary is the amount of simple carbohydrate, and this will be noted in the appropriate section. You can also modify your meal timing if intermittent fasting (I.F.; two meals per day) is one of your recommendations. For certain gene coding, this will not be ideal, for example FTO (AA) and MC4R (CC) but is possible if you find

I.F. hard to follow. However, you must move to only three meals a day with no snacking at all. You must leave five to six hours between meals.

Supplements are also a place where dosing often changes at the eight-week mark. As with diet, once your genes and your metabolism are working optimally, supplements can be reduced or discontinued. Instructions are included for each gene in the treatment plan.

Natural Supplements

The natural supplements recommended in my treatment protocols are not essential but will greatly improve your response and outcome. For many individuals, poor dietary habits will have resulted in metabolic and genetic changes that can be difficult to reverse with diet alone, which is why I incorporate supplements as part of the program for my patients. In addition, supplements can make the transition period of genetic retraining much easier and can target secondary issues such as chronic stress, which can be more difficult to control.

Supplements are available through your health-care practitioner or directly through health stores, Amazon or www.thisisgoodmedicine.com.

Before starting any supplement program, I recommend you discuss them with your health-care practitioner.

Weight Loss

With respect to weight loss, there will certainly be those of you that wish to use your genetic profile to help achieve or maintain a healthy body mass, and the recommendations will certainly offer plenty of advice in that area. However, many will just wish to improve their overall health in terms of reducing diabetes or hyperlipidemia risk, increasing energy levels and staying fit. Treatment sections will include advice for those individuals too, either as part of a general plan or in a separate "weight-stable" section.

Selected SNPs

The gene SNPs included in this book are the following:

FTO

FTO, the Fat Mass and Obesity-Related Protein gene, originally known as the "fatso" gene because of its large size, codes for the enzyme alpha-ketoglutarate-dependent dioxygenase. It was one of the first metabolic genes identified, and research into its clinical and lifestyle implications is extensive. It has a significant impact on hunger and satiety through effects on hormones such as ghrelin and leptin. Through its influence on production of the hormone adiponectin, it affects insulin sensitivity, fatty acid oxidation, the regulation of glucose and insulin levels, and the amount and type of fat storage. Although diet, exercise and lifestyle exert influence over a number of metabolic genes, their impact on the FTO SNP is particularly profound and provides significant treatment avenues for the management of variability within this gene.

ADIPOQ

The ADIPOQ gene codes for the 244-amino acid protein adiponectin, circulating in high concentrations in the blood of normal individuals. Adiponectin is a bioactive, fat cell–derived hormone (adipokine) produced primarily in adipose tissue. There is some production in bone marrow, the cardiovascular system, the liver and muscle mass, but it is produced in highest concentration in fatty tissue. It increases insulin sensitivity, at least partially, by suppressing glucose production, increases fatty acid oxidation and regulates glucose and insulin levels. It increases healthy fat storage while preventing accumulation of lipids in other tissues (liver, muscle and arteries, among others) and has a strong cardio-protective role. Treatment is aimed at increasing adiponectin levels, adjusting dietary intake to mitigate any effects of low adiponectin and reducing cortisol, which, as we have seen, further impairs adiponectin production. Besides improving weight management, optimizing adiponectin has the potential to reduce long-term risk of insulin resistance and type 2 diabetes. It may also prove beneficial in terms of vascular disease and obesity-related cancers.

MC4R

The MC4R gene codes for the Melanocortin-4 Receptor in the hypothalamus of the brain. This receptor has a central role in satiety and controlled food intake. When stimulated by the agonist neuropeptide α-MSH (alpha melanocyte stimulating hormone), it reduces hunger, improves sensitivity to satiety signals, promotes meal termination and increases metabolism, fat burning and thermogenesis. Therefore, the MC4 receptor plays a pivotal role in the tonic control of food intake, energy expenditure and weight homeostasis. The variant C-allele is associated with an increase in BMI of 0.22 kg/m^2 and the homozygote variant CC can increase body weight by up to 43% independent of diet and exercise. It is associated with a tendency to gravitate to energy-dense foods and with emotional or stress-related eating. Individuals with the risk allele benefit greatly from restricted calorie intake and intermittent fasting.

PPARG

PPARG is a complex gene working through numerous mechanisms. It has an important role in glucose and fat metabolism, insulin sensitivity and inflammation. The variant G-allele is associated with improved insulin sensitivity and a *reduced* risk of developing type 2 diabetes *in normal-weight individuals*. The PPAR-gamma or glitazone receptor is the target for the TZD (thiazolidinediones) class of diabetic medications, which work by stimulating the PPARG receptor to increase adipogenesis and fatty acid uptake by peripheral tissues. The resulting decrease in fatty acid availability improves insulin sensitivity. The gene product has several different functions and has been coined the master regulator of adipocyte biology. It works by modifying the transcription of a number of genes involved in glucose and lipid metabolism, fat cell differentiation and energy balance. It also has an anti-inflammatory effect on the endothelial cells that line the cardiovascular system and reduces the development of atherosclerosis. Although the variant allele (G) may confer some health benefits, its expression is highly sensitive to diet and exercise. A diet low in saturated fat and carbohydrates along with endurance exercise are essential to maintain the beneficial effects of the allele.

APOA2

The APOA2 gene encodes for Apolipoprotein A2, which is the second most abundant high-density lipoprotein in the body. Apolipoproteins A1 and A2 are the major protein components of high-density lipoproteins or HDLs, the "good cholesterol" that removes excess bad cholesterol from the blood and reduces atherosclerosis and cardiovascular disease risk. It plays a significant role in modulating the body's response to dietary saturated fat. The association between the variant allele of the APOA2 gene, high BMI and a high-fat diet is one of the strongest examples of nutrigenomics, that is, the interaction of diet with gene expression. A mean increase in BMI of 6.2% is seen in CC versus CT or TT individuals when consuming equally high amounts of saturated fat exceeding 22 grams per day. This association is of particular importance in societies with abundant food and food high in fat content (such as a typical western diet).

FABP2

Fatty Acid Binding Protein 2 is one of a group of proteins that play a key role in the absorption and intracellular transport of long-chain fatty acids. It is produced primarily in the small intestine and encoded by the FABP2 gene. A-allele carriers (homozygous AA or heterozygous GA) are far more likely to have increased serum glucose levels both after fasting and after a large meal rich in saturated fats and sugars. In addition, the amount of saturated fat consumed appears to have a profound effect on the phenotype expressed in A-allele individuals. Those that eat a diet containing 53 grams or more of saturated fat per day have a lower HDL-to-total cholesterol ratio; higher cholesterol, LDLs and triglycerides; and higher insulin resistance. Overweight or obese adults with the A-allele that followed a low-calorie, low-saturated-fat diet for one month had significantly lower C-reactive protein, smaller waist circumference and lower waist-to-hip ratio when compared to GG genotypes. So although the variant allele increases risk, carriers respond more positively to dietary changes than those with the wild allele G.

TCF7L2

TCF7L2 or TransCription Factor 7-Like 2 codes for the protein T-cell transcription factor 4 (TCF4) and is highly implicated in blood glucose homeostasis. It alters the expression of other genes that control insulin after the consumption of carbohydrates and saturated fats. The SNP rs7903146 is one of two SNPs linked with TCF7L2, the other being rs4506565. They are both strongly implicated in the development of type 2 diabetes with a correlation of 92%. The SNP rs7903146 is the stronger of the two in terms of etiological association. The T-allele is strongly linked to the development of type 2 diabetes across multiple populations. Numerous studies have demonstrated the SNP increases population-attributable risk by 16 to 21%. Heterozygous individuals have a Relative Risk of 1.45 while the homozygous genotype confers a Relative Risk of 2.41.

IRS1

The gene IRS1 codes for the protein Insulin Receptor Substrate 1, which plays a key role in the insulin receptor signal transduction pathway and the cellular effects of insulin. Along with other SNPs at the same IRS1 gene locus, the rs2943641 variant allele is associated with an increased ratio of visceral to subcutaneous fat, insulin resistance, metabolic syndrome, poor lipid profile, and increased risk of type 2 diabetes and coronary artery disease. The risk allele (C) is associated with increased deposition of visceral fat, insulin resistance and an increase in type 2 diabetes risk of up to 20%. A diet low in high-glycemic carbohydrates and saturated fats significantly reduces the risk.

The Stress Genes (ADRB2, NR3C2, CRHR1, FKBP5)

The importance and pervasiveness of chronic stress within our society is unarguable and its role in the development and progression of disease increasingly recognized (see *The Complete Doctor's Stress*

Solution by Dr. Penny Kendall-Reed and Dr. Stephen Reed, Publisher Robert Rose, 2004, *ISBN 0-7788-0096-2*). The impact of stress on energy utilization, body weight, food craving and metabolic disease has been an important part of my clinical practice for many years so its role in genetics was the next piece of the puzzle. That is why I have included these SNPs in my program and this book.

The rapidly expanding field of epigenetics examines how modification of genetic expression—rather than genetic code—can influence health and disease. Lifestyle factors such as diet and exercise can modify transcription of certain genes by enzymatically attaching a chemical tag (most commonly a methyl group). Epigenetic tags can be added or deleted through generations. One factor that exerts a profound influence on gene expression is chronic stress, with new research indicating that alterations in function may be inheritable.

The importance of stress in the expression of variant genotypes is extremely important. For example, despite ideal SNP coding for genes TCF7L2 and IRS1, increased cortisol will triple the release of insulin to carbohydrates such as grains, starches, sweets and fruits, forcing the body to treat one apple as the equivalent of three apples or one cookie as a whole box! In one study looking at the association of the variant MC4R C-allele with obesity, once adjusted for other variables, the results indicated that those individuals with high stress levels had a stronger association with higher BMI and preferential intake of processed and fat-dense foods over fruits and vegetables.

Chapter 5 Metabolic Gene Summary Table

FTO	The Fat Mass and Obesity-related Protein ("fatso gene")	• Profound impact on hunger and satiety through its effects on signalling hormones • Risk allele increases body mass by 1% and obesity risk by 22% • Highly modifiable by diet, exercise and lifestyle	Risk = A Ideal = T
ADIPOQ (2 SNPs)	Codes for the fat cell hormone adiponectin	• Modulates glucose and insulin and increases fat mobilization • Increases insulin sensitivity • Reduces unhealthy fat storage • Risk alleles have a significant impact on ability to lose weight	rs17366568 Risk = A Ideal = G rs17300539 Risk = G Ideal = A
MC4R	Codes for the melanocortin-4 receptor in the brain	• Central role in hunger and satiety signalling • Reduces feelings of hunger and craving • Important control over food intake • Risk allele associated with body weight increase of up to 43%	Risk = C Ideal = T
PPARG	PPAR-gamma or glitazone receptor gene	• Important role in glucose and fat metabolism • Affects insulin sensitivity and inflammation • Highly sensitive to diet and exercise	Risk = C Ideal = G

Gene	Function	Details	Alleles
APOA2	Codes for the "good cholesterol" component apolipoprotein A2	• Removes bad cholesterol and reduces vascular disease risk • Modulates the body's response to dietary fat • Risk allele increases body mass by 6.2% • Strongly influenced by diet	Risk = C Ideal = T
FABP2	Fatty acid binding protein plays a strong role in the absorption and metabolism of fats	• Affects sensitivity to dietary fats and sugar • Risk allele has twice the affinity for dietary fat • Risk allele increases diabetes risk • Highly sensitive to diet	Risk = A Ideal = G
TCF7L2	Codes for T-cell transcription factor 4 and highly implicated in blood sugar control	• Alters the activity of genes controlling insulin release • Risk allele strongly implicated in the development of type 2 diabetes • Strongly influenced by diet	Risk = T Ideal = C
IRS1	Codes for insulin receptor substrate 1 affecting insulin and glucose control	• Controls glucose uptake and metabolism • Risk allele associated with insulin resistance and increased diabetes probability by up to 21% • Modified by dietary carbohydrate and fat	Risk = C Ideal = T

GeneRx.ca

GeneRx.ca is my online platform that allows your health-care practitioner or licensed fitness expert to upload your raw 23andMe SNP data and obtain a personalized health analysis and treatment protocol. Other genetic platforms only provide interpretation of single gene SNPs. They offer incomplete, hard-to-follow and often-conflicting information and advice. *GeneRx.ca* uses my own clinically developed algorithms to analyze combinations of genes, providing a more detailed, comprehensive and individualized report. Only by considering the complex interactions between multiple genes can a truly personalized and effective profile be presented.

The following are SNP category examples from *GeneRx.ca*:

Metabolic: MC4R, ADIPOQ, FTO, PPARG, ADRB2
This section looks at the production of and sensitivity to the three main hormones adiponectin, leptin and ghrelin, which control the rate of metabolism, satiety, hunger and food cravings. It also looks at how the central nervous system impacts lipogenesis, the formation of fat from food, as well as examining the genetic influence on thermogenesis. Finally, it identifies which individuals have a metabolism that functions best with intermittent fasting or three meals a day. It creates an individualized protocol to maximize metabolic function helping to prevent and treat weight gain and obesity, diabetes and unstable blood sugar levels.

Carbohydrate Handling: IRS1, GIPR, TCF7L2
This section looks at the production of and sensitivity to the three main hormones adiponectin, leptin and ghrelin, which control the rate of the metabolism, satiety, hunger and food cravings. It also looks at how the central nervous system impacts lipogenesis, the formation of fat form food, as well as examining the genetic influence on thermogenesis. Finally, it identifies which individuals have a metabolism that functions best with intermittent fasting or three meals a day. It creates an individualized protocol to maximize metabolic function helping to prevent and treat weight gain and obesity, diabetes and unstable blood sugar levels.

Fat Handling: FTO, APOA2, FABP2
This section looks at how saturated fats can affect the production and response to the three metabolic hormones leptin, adiponectin and

ghrelin. It explains how fats can influence weight gain and alter satiety and food-seeking behaviour. It shows who has a decreased ability to break down stored fat on the body, who increases LDL production and who produces more inflammatory substrates when consuming saturated fats. This section will then provide the exact gram content of recommended saturated fats per day to help prevent high cholesterol and obesity. A table of saturated fat content in foods to help guide better dietary choices will also be provided.

What Is Different about a GeneRx.ca Report?

Compared to a typical report available online, the GeneRx.ca report not only looks at how genes influence each other but also provides far more detailed and comprehensive information along with treatment protocols. As an example, consider the three major genes controlling carbohydrate response, TCF7L2, IRS1 and GIPR.

A Typical Report:
This report would look at the three genes individually and provide minimal guidance.

TCF7L2 – Variant or red – you do not respond well to carbohydrates and need to restrict them.

IRS1 – Normal or green – you do respond well to carbohydrates, and you do not need to restrict them.

GIPR – Heterozygote or yellow – you respond less well to carbohydrates, and you need to moderate your carbohydrate consumption.

A GeneRx Report:
This report looks at all three genes together and clearly explains what it means to respond well or poorly. It provides an individualized carbohydrate count and dietary protocol based on the integration of the three genes.

TCF7L2 – TT = Variant
IRS1 – TT = Normal
GIPR – CT = Heterozygote

You are very sensitive to carbohydrates. You make more insulin and inflammatory substrates to carbohydrates, destabilizing blood sugars, increasing inflammation particularly in the bowel and stomach, and increasing weight gain more easily upon carbohydrate consumption.

Keep grains, starches, fruits or alcohol (see list of carbohydrates to moderate below) to a maximum of two meals per day for eight weeks, where the physical size of the carbohydrate is half the physical size of the protein. Do not use sweets as your carbohydrate on a regular basis; save that as a treat.

Keep healthy vegetables such as broccoli, zucchini, peppers and cauliflower as your main carbohydrate source. You can consume unlimited quantities of these vegetables and salads, avoiding the starchy ones below.

Carbohydrates to moderate:
Grains: breads, pastas, rice, corn, popcorn, quinoa, legumes, muffins, crackers
Starches: potato, sweet potato, yam, squash, carrot, beets, turnip
Fruits: all fruits except tomatoes; berries are the best choice
Alcohol: wine, spirits, beer
Sweets: cakes, pastries, cookies, candy, soda pop, hot chocolate

Supplements:
Metabolic Xtra by Pure Encapsulations or Berb-Evail by Designs for Health: one capsule 30 minutes before meals for eight weeks if blood sugars are unstable

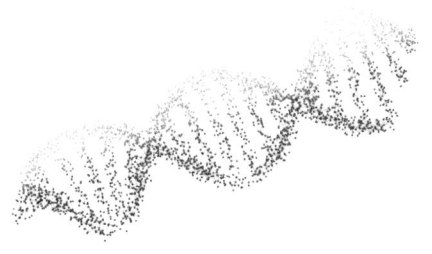

CHAPTER 7
Case Study # 3
Transition-Years Diet

Mary, a 29-year-old female, had been gaining weight fairly steadily since finishing university. In the past six years, she had gained 53 pounds. In the first year of weight gain, she had not changed her diet significantly, but "probably ate more grains and starches" than when she lived at home. She had been vegan for many years, eating a great deal of legumes, tofu, nuts, seeds, grains, vegan cheeses and yogurts, vegetables and fruits. She ate no dairy, wheat, direct sugars or animal products. She did not consume coconut oil products or medium-chain triglycerides (MCT) due to the saturated-fat content.

Discouraged by her weight gain, she further "tightened" up her diet, changing her vegan dairy substitute products to lower fat and reducing portions at each meal. She began slipping into a mild depression, with low energy and poor motivation.

Mary's genetic profile included the following coding:

- FTO: TT – normal metabolic rate
- PPARG: CC – weight gain worse with high-fat, high-carbohydrate diet
- TCF7L2: TT – increased glucose and insulin response to carbohydrates

- IRS1: TC – increased glucose and insulin response to carbohydrates
- APOA2: TT – low risk of increased LDL, weight gain or inflammation with more than 22 grams of saturated fat
- FABP2: GG – low risk of weight gain with saturated fats

In our late 20s and early 30s, we go through what are called transition years. This is where the body "stops growing and starts aging." There is a significant shift in enzyme and hormone production, cellular turnover and repair. During these years (as well as our menopausal/andropausal years, our second set of transition years), genetic expression can increase or decrease. This is what has occurred with Mary. She is not designed to consume a great deal of carbohydrates as determined by her TCF7L2, IRS1 and PPARG genes. Similarly, she does very well with fats, both saturated and unsaturated. And in fact, a low-fat diet will decrease her dopamine production leading to food cravings, low moods and most of all decreased motivation.

Based on her genetics, I recommended the following protocol:

- Increased fats in her diet. I recommended predominantly unsaturated fats from nuts, seeds and avocados but also advised she could increase her saturated fats to approximately 30 to 35 grams per day if she wished. As she is vegan, her saturated fats were predominantly in the form of nuts, seeds, coconut oil, MCT oils and full-fat vegan diary alternatives.
- I reduced her protein to 0.7 grams of protein per kilogram of body weight per day, divided between her three meals.
- I advised she have carbohydrates in the form of grains, fruit, starches, sweets or alcohol at only one meal per day, where the physical size of that carbohydrate was ½ the physical size of the protein.
- Vegetables and salads were unlimited.
- No supplements needed

Results

Despite being very reluctant to move away from her low-fat, high "healthy" carb diet, she decided to give this a try. In the first week, she lost two pounds and continued to lose an average of two pounds per week for the next 23 weeks for a total loss of 46 pounds. Within two weeks, she felt energetic, with better mood throughout the day, and her motivation for life returned. She eventually stabilized her weight, having lost 58 pounds to achieve a level she was very happy with. Mary found the diet easy to follow and continued with it long term to maximize her health. At two and a half years, her health and energy are excellent, and her weight remains stable.

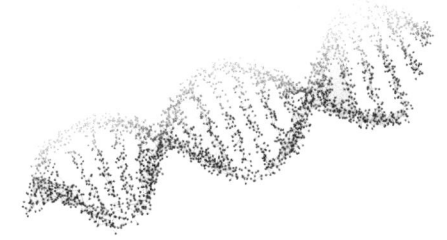

GUIDE TO GENE CHAPTERS

The following chapters highlight specific gene SNPs. If you have completed a DNA analysis and know your personal coding for these SNPs then this might be a good time to take note of them. That way you can refer to the sections most relevant to you. For each gene you will find a summary of the risk allele attributes (Quick Look), background information and research about the gene along with treatment protocols for each possible SNP coding. There may also be information on its interaction with other genes. To find your individual protocol, look for the treatment section with your allele coding.

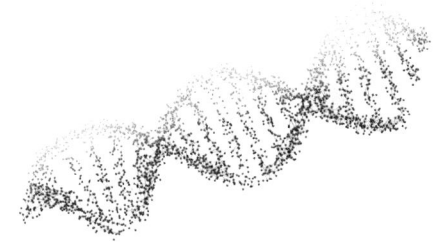

CHAPTER 8
FTO

The Fat Mass and Obesity Gene
rs9939609
Normal/Ancestral allele – T
Variant/Risk allele – A

FTO Quick Look

FTO A-allele (risk)
- *Increased production of ghrelin, the "hunger hormone," decreased post-prandial suppression of ghrelin and greater hypothalamic sensitivity to ghrelin*
- *Reduced leptin sensitivity (leptin resistance). Leptin is the "satiety hormone," reducing hunger and food-seeking behaviour. Leptin resistance leads to an inability to mobilize and use fat stores and is associated with cravings, typically late evening and overnight*
- *Decreased adiponectin leading to poor insulin sensitivity. Decreased fatty acid oxidation and impaired regulation of glucose and insulin levels*
- *Slower metabolism and impaired fat burning*
- *Increased white fat production*

FTO T-allele (normal)
- *No associated risk; ideal coding*

FTO, the Fat Mass and Obesity-Related Gene (also known as the "fatso" gene), codes for the enzyme alpha-ketoglutarate-dependent dioxygenase. It was one of the first metabolic genes identified, and research into its clinical and lifestyle implications is extensive.

FTO codes for an enzyme involved in DNA and RNA methylation and is therefore able to influence the expression of other genes. The precise mechanism by which FTO works is not fully understood, but it appears to have a profound effect on the control of hunger and satiety, greatly affecting food intake and eating behaviour. Research has found high levels of FTO gene expression in areas of the hypothalamus known to be responsible for the regulation of metabolism, energy intake and expenditure, and hunger-satiety modulation. Hypothalamic FTO expression is also shown to be modulated by fasting. In addition, it influences energy homeostasis, fat storage and insulin sensitivity through its effect on the fat hormone adiponectin and the fat cell differentiation proteins IRX-3 and IRX-5 (see below for further information on these hormones).

Appetite or hunger is described as the desire to search for food, eat or keep eating, while satiety is the sensation of being full, which leads to diminished food-seeking behaviour and intake. Those with high satiety lose their appetite towards the end of a meal while individuals with a *low-satiety* response remain hungry and continue to seek out and consume food even after eating a meal. They also have a tendency to gravitate toward energy-dense foods containing sugars and fats. The control systems for appetite reside in the hypothalamus of the brain and are influenced both by local neurochemical inputs and by feedback from peripherally released hormones.

There is a balance between the "hunger centre" and the "satiety centre," both located in the hypothalamus (see Figure 1). The hunger centre in the lateral hypothalamus stimulates feeding behaviour and energy storage through chemical mediators such as MCH (Melanin Concentrating Hormone), the Orexins and the Cannabinoid system. The satiety centre in the ventromedial hypothalamus leads to reduced hunger and food-seeking and increased energy expenditure via the melanocortin pathway (MC4 receptors).

Figure 1: Hunger and Satiety interactions in the hypothalamus

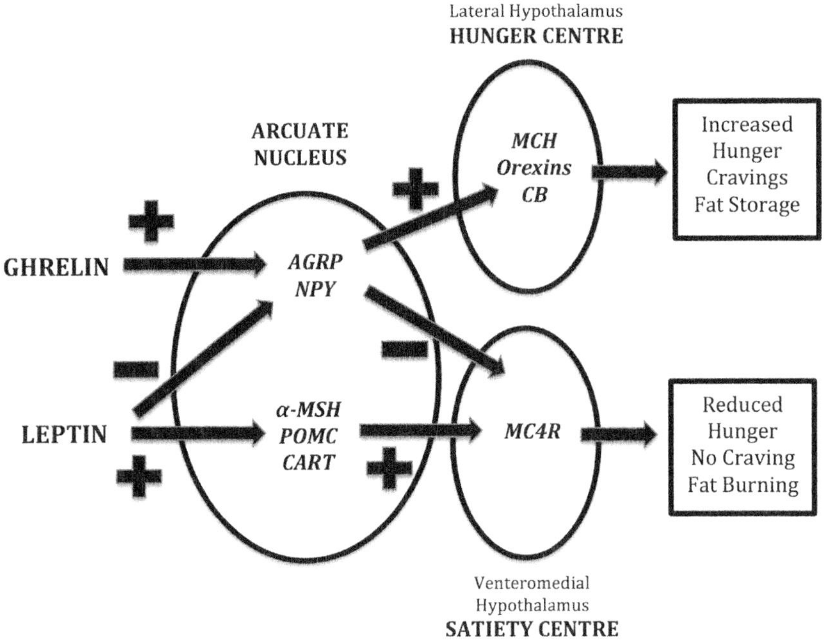

```
                          Lateral Hypothalamus
                            HUNGER CENTRE

           ARCUATE                                    Increased
           NUCLEUS         MCH                        Hunger
                          Orexins         →           Cravings
                            CB                        Fat Storage
    +              +

GHRELIN  →      AGRP
                NPY
                                   —
    —

LEPTIN   →     α-MSH                                  Reduced
               POMC          MC4R         →           Hunger
               CART                                   No Craving
                     +                                Fat Burning

                           Venteromedial
                           Hypothalamus
                          SATIETY CENTRE
```

AGRP	Agouti-related peptide
NPY	Neuropeptide-Y
MCH	Melanin Concentrating Hormone
CB	Cannabinoid System
α-MSH	Alpha-Melanocyte Stimulating Hormone
POMC	Propriomelanocortin
CART	Cocaine and amphetamine related transcript
+	**Stimulates**
—	**Inhibits**

The brain is "hardwired to be hungry." The primary drive is from AGRP and NPY, which stimulate the hunger centre and turn off the satiety centre. We need adequate hormonal messages from the body such as leptin to turn this drive off.

The overwhelming drive within our brain is to seek out and consume food. In effect, we are "hardwired to be hungry." The arcuate nucleus constantly drives the "hunger centre" and inhibits the "satiety centre," leading to food-seeking behaviour and cravings while promoting fat storage. It is not until sufficient satiety feedback messages are received (such as leptin) that the balance shifts. The "hunger" chemicals (AGRP and NPY) are switched off and the satiety chemicals (α-MSH, POMC and CART) released, switching on the satiety centre, reducing hunger and cravings, and promoting fat burning. It is not surprising that disruption to this satiety feedback mechanism results in significant overeating. The two most important peripheral hormones influencing this system are leptin and ghrelin. Increased leptin actively shuts off the hunger centre while stimulating the satiety centre. Ghrelin on the other hand is a strong stimulator of the hunger centre, so reducing its concentration is essential to mitigate its effects and allow the satiety centre to influence behaviour.

Ghrelin
Ghrelin, our hunger hormone (also known as Lenomorelin) is a peptide hormone produced in the gastrointestinal tract. It functions as a chemical messenger, or neuropeptide, in the central nervous system to regulate appetite. Unlike many biochemical messengers, ghrelin is easily able to cross the blood-brain barrier, giving rise to its powerful impact on central hunger control.

When the stomach is empty and fuel stores are low, such as after several hours of not eating, ghrelin is released to direct the brain (hunger/satiety centres in the hypothalamus) to seek out food for fuel and help co-ordinate the use of energy in the body. Ghrelin also acts locally in the gastrointestinal tract by increasing the release of gastric acid and stimulating gastrointestinal motility. This is done to prepare the body for incoming food. After a meal, or when the stomach is stretched, production and secretion of ghrelin is stopped.

In the brain, ghrelin binds to the ghrelin-growth hormone secretagogue receptor (GHSR) in the arcuate nucleus, increasing the release of the protein agouti-related peptide (AgRP). AgRP inhibits the MC4R (melanocortin-4 receptor) in the satiety centre (ventromedial hypothalamus), turning it off. At the same time, it stimulates activity in the hunger centre (lateral hypothalamus) by increasing MCH, Orexin and CB activity.

Ghrelin also plays an important role in the perception of reward from food. This is mediated through its stimulation of dopamine-releasing neurons within the ventral tegmental area of the brain, which connects to the nucleus accumbens. The nucleus accumbens is the area that processes desire and reward, reinforcing addictive behaviour.

Leptin
Leptin is the "satiety hormone," reducing hunger and food-seeking behaviour. It gives the brain an "I'm full" message. Released by fat cells, it crosses into the brain and acts on the POMC/CART neurons of the arcuate nucleus, causing them to release the neurotransmitter α-MSH. α-MSH binds to and stimulates the MC4 receptor in the satiety centre, reducing the sensation of hunger and increasing metabolism. Peripherally, leptin decreases lipogenesis (the formation of fatty adipose tissue) and increases adipose tissue breakdown through triglyceride (TG) hydrolysis and fatty acid oxidation. Acting through the sympathetic nervous system, it acts on brown and white fat to increase metabolism and promote lipolysis. Leptin resistance leads to an inability to mobilize and use fat stores and is associated with cravings, typically late evening and overnight.

Unfortunately, the satiety factors that appear most influenced by FTO are leptin and ghrelin. The A-allele, for example, is associated with *increased* production of ghrelin, which causes increased food cravings, particularly for energy-dense foods such as sugars and fats. It is also associated with *reduced* leptin sensitivity or "leptin resistance." In this condition, the receptors in the arcuate nucleus become insensitive to leptin, and the ability of this hormone to switch off the hunger centre and stimulate the satiety centre becomes markedly impaired.

Adiponectin

FTO also affects the hormone adiponectin, produced primarily in our fat cells. There is some production in bone marrow, the cardiovascular system, the liver and muscle mass, but it is produced in highest concentration in adipose tissue. It increases insulin sensitivity, increases fatty acid oxidation and regulates glucose and insulin levels. It increases healthy fat storage while preventing accumulation of lipids in other tissues (liver, muscle and arteries, among others) and has a strong cardio-protective role. Reduced fat mass *increases* adiponectin, which promotes glucose and fatty acid uptake into adipocytes. Adiponectin reduces the production of cholesterol and glucose by the liver so helps control metabolic syndrome. Overall it has a profound effect on the storage and use of fat as an energy source.

Genetic abnormalities causing lowered adiponectin levels result in obesity, insulin resistance, type 2 diabetes and metabolic syndrome. The paradox of a hormone that is produced by fat cells yet shows *decreased* levels in obesity is explained in part by the finding that adiponectin secretion by fat cells is *inversely* proportional to their size (diameter). In effect, obesity leads to dysfunctional fat cells that are no longer able to function effectively in controlling energy storage and metabolism. There is some evidence that the A-allele leads to reduced expression of the adiponectin gene in fat cells and therefore contributes to this functional deterioration.

IRX Proteins

Research into the mechanism by which the FTO gene affects adiposity has revealed an important interaction with two protein sequences that affect fat cell development. These proteins, IRX-3 and IRX-5 (Iroquois-class homeodomain proteins 3 and 5), induce progenitor fat cells to form white fat cells rather than brown fat cells. White fat is considered "bad" and is associated with the ill effects of obesity, while brown or thermogenic fat (BAT) actually increases metabolism, burns fatty acids and improves glucose metabolism. The normal FTO gene product (T-allele) reduces levels of IRX-3 and -5 in adipocytes via the repressor protein ARID5B, thereby promoting development into BAT. Individuals with the variant A-allele have impairment of ARID5B binding and therefore a markedly reduced ability to exert this beneficial effect on their adipocytes compared to those with the normal T-allele. In some studies, this effect is shown to be by a factor of five times.

In one research study (Claussnitzer, 2015), the gene-editing method CRISPR-Cas9 was used on adipocyte precursor cells to convert their obesity-promoting FTO risk variant (A) to the normal variant (T). The treated cells had significantly lowered levels of IRX-3 and IRX-5, converted to brown adipocytes and increased their metabolism sevenfold.

FTO SNP rs9939609
Normal/Ancestral allele – T
Variant/Risk allele – A

The prevalence of the risk allele (A) varies greatly between populations. Chinese and Japanese individuals show the lowest prevalence (2% for AA and 25% for AT), while in Kenya these values are 35% and 47%, respectively. Overall, in large-scale multiple population studies, the risk allele accounts for an overall 1% increase in the body mass index (BMI) and a 22% increased risk of obesity, *independent* of diet and exercise. However, the effect is significantly worse if an FTO-A individual consumes a low-protein, high-*saturated* fat or high-calorie diet. In an example of nutritional epigenetics, the influence of the A-allele is greatly enhanced with such nutrition. In a striking illustration of this effect, the FTO A-allele has a prevalence of over 75% in some African populations yet the incidence of obesity and diabetes is extremely low as a result of their low-fat diet. Individuals of African descent living in the United States and consuming a typical western high-saturated-fat diet have a similar prevalence of FTO-A but much higher BMI and type 2 diabetes risk.

The A-allele is associated with the following:
- Increased production of ghrelin, the "hunger hormone," decreased post-prandial suppression of ghrelin and greater hypothalamic sensitivity to ghrelin; an association with binge eating
- Reduced leptin sensitivity (leptin resistance). Leptin is the "satiety hormone," reducing hunger and food-seeking behaviour. Leptin decreases lipogenesis and increases TG hydrolysis and fatty acid oxidation. Acting through the sympathetic nervous system, it acts on brown and white fat to increase metabolism and promote lipolysis. Leptin resistance leads to an inability to mobilize and use fat stores and is associated with cravings, typically late evening and overnight.
- Decreased adiponectin. Adiponectin increases insulin sensitivity, increases fatty acid oxidation and regulates glucose and insulin levels. It increases healthy fat storage while preventing accumulation of lipids in other tissues (liver, muscle and arteries, among others) and has a strong cardio-protective role. Adiponectin reduces the production of cholesterol and glucose by the liver so helps control metabolic syndrome. Overall, it has a profound effect on the storage and use of fat as an energy source.
- Increased white fat adipogenesis through its effect on IRX-3 and IRX-5
- Slower metabolism secondary to leptin resistance, decreased adiponectin and less brown fat
- Impaired fat burning

There is a large amount of data supporting the association of the risk allele (A) with higher BMI, obesity, diabetes and metabolic syndrome, with the allele exerting its greatest influence through the desire to consume energy-dense foods. Adults with the variant risk allele (A) tend to consume, on average, 125 to 280 more calories per day than do T-allele carriers. The overall effect of the A-allele is quite profound, with heterozygote (TA) carriers weighing an average 1.2 kilograms (2.6 pounds) more than TT individuals. Homozygote (AA) carriers weigh an average 3 kilograms (6.6 pounds) more than TT individuals and have 1.67 times the risk of obesity compared to TT individuals. This rises to 2.5 times if ingesting a high-carbohydrate or high-fat diet. The trend is seen as early as age seven and continues throughout life (Sandholt, 2012).

Frayling (2007) found, in the population he studied, that 16% of adults who were homozygous for the risk allele weighed about 3 kilograms more and had 1.67-fold increased odds of obesity when compared with those not inheriting a risk allele. This association was observed from age seven years upward and reflected a specific increase in fat mass.

Appetite or hunger is described as the desire to search for food, eat or keep eating, while satiety is the sensation of being full, which leads to diminished food-seeking behaviour and intake. Those with high satiety lose their appetite towards the end of a meal while individuals with a *low-satiety* response remain hungry and continue to seek out and consume food even after eating a meal. They also have a tendency to gravitate toward energy-dense foods containing sugars and fats. A study from 2013 (Karra, 2013) on normal-weight subjects found A-allele carriers to have higher levels of ghrelin and impaired suppression of this hunger hormone after a meal. Their brains were more sensitive to the effect of ghrelin, and their reward pathways had increased response to food images on functional magnetic resonance imaging (MRI). Elevated ghrelin levels are, at least in part, the result of reduced methylation of ghrelin mRNA and likely a direct result of the biochemical influence of the FTO gene product.

Most studies show that the A-allele is associated with higher leptin levels, which would seem inconsistent with what we know about their phenotype; higher BMIs; and feeling hungrier and eating more than individuals with a T-allele. This paradox is likely explained by an increased level of leptin *resistance* in both the hypothalamus and peripheral tissues in those carrying the variant allele. Leptin resistance leads to an inability to mobilize and use fat stores and is associated with cravings, typically late evening and overnight.

Adiponectin (which is also discussed in the next chapter in terms of its own gene polymorphisms) is a hormone produced primarily in our fat cells. Overall, it has a profound effect on the storage and use of fat as an energy source. Genetic abnormalities causing lowered adiponectin levels result in obesity, insulin resistance, type 2 diabetes and metabolic syndrome. The paradox of a hormone that is produced by fat cells yet shows *decreased* levels in obesity is explained in part by the finding that adiponectin secretion by fat cells is *inversely* proportional to their size (diameter). In effect, obesity leads to dysfunctional fat cells that are no longer able to function effectively in controlling energy storage and metabolism. There is some evidence that the A-allele leads to reduced expression of the adiponectin gene in fat cells and therefore contributes to this functional deterioration.

Obesity is directly related to the ability of fat cells to increase in size and store fat beyond their normal capacity. This leads to insulin resistance and inflammation. Research into the mechanism by which the FTO gene affects adiposity has revealed an important interaction with two protein sequences that affect fat cell development. These proteins, IRX-3 and IRX-5 (Iroquois-class homeodomain proteins 3 and 5), induce progenitor fat cells to form white fat cells rather than brown fat cells (BAT or brown adipose tissue). White adipose tissue is the unhealthy storage form of fat, while brown adipose tissue is a metabolically active form that actually burns fat to create heat. Individuals with higher levels of BAT have a higher metabolic rate, burn more calories and tend to be leaner. The normal FTO gene product (T-allele) reduces levels of IRX-3 and -5 in adipocytes via the repressor protein ARID5B, thereby promoting development of BAT. Individuals with the variant A-allele have impairment of ARID5B binding, which decreases this beneficial effect by a factor of five times.

The overall effect of leptin resistance, low adiponectin and altered fat cell metabolism (increased white fat, decreased brown fat and impaired fat burning) is to reduce overall metabolic rate. This, coupled with the increased intake of energy-dense foods, can result in unwanted weight gain.

Impact of Activity

Although important for a number of metabolic genes, the impact of diet, exercise and lifestyle on disease risk associated with FTO SNPs is quite profound and provides significant treatment avenues for management of genetic variability. Increased calorific intake and low exercise levels are shown to have a strongly additive effect on the risk of obesity and diabetes associated with the A-allele. In one study (Ahmad, 2011), the *increase* in BMI per risk allele varied between 0.22 kg/m^2 for active individuals consuming a low-calorie diet to 0.97 kg/m^2 for those that were inactive with high-calorific intake. Obesity risk increased in a similar manner, and there was also a significant increase in the risk of type 2 diabetes with higher food intake and low exercise. (Note that this study looked at the FTO SNP rs8050136, a SNP with similar A-allele variant phenotype that is in complete linkage disequilibrium with rs9939609, meaning it correlates with regards to population disease risk.) Although the A-allele tends to increase BMI and risk of obesity, Ahmad's research illustrates how diet and exercise can exert epigenetic control over its expression. Results are summarized in the following table.

	Regular Exercise		Inactive	
	Low Calorie	High Calorie	Low Calorie	High Calorie
Increase in Obesity Risk (per A-allele)	1.13	1.15	1.21	1.39
BMI Difference (kg/m^2)	+0.22	+0.38	+0.49	+0.97

(From Ahmad, 2011)

The association between low activity level and increased phenotype expression of the FTO A-allele has been demonstrated in numerous studies indicating that physical activity may go some way to counteracting the effects of the risk allele. The same is true for higher calorie intake. Other studies have indicated that dietary content may also play a significant role in the expression of the SNP. A high intake of saturated fats was found to significantly increase the risk of high BMI in North American carriers of the FTO risk allele (Corella, 2011).

The role of the FTO SNPs in obesity, satiety and metabolic dysfunction continues to expand as a better understanding of its numerous interactions is explored. There remains some conflicting research, which may be explained by the interaction of FTO with other genes and SNPs and the populations under study. Magno's study, for example, found lower ghrelin and higher leptin in AA individuals (Magno, 2018). However, the population studied was morbidly obese and therefore represented the "end stage" effect of genetic influence and lifestyle choices. The metabolic alterations that have occurred at this point are profound, making interpretation in terms of pre-disease individuals difficult.

TREATMENT

FTO The Fat Mass and Obesity Gene, rs9939609
Normal/Ancestral allele – T
Variant/Risk allele – A

FTO is a gene that responds dramatically to changes in diet and exercise. Reference to the table above (from Ahmad, 2011) shows that incorporating exercise and a low-calorie diet can reduce the BMI increase associated with the A-allele from 0.97 kg/m^2 to 0.22 kg/m^2. The increased obesity risk can similarly be reduced from 1.39 to 1.13.

Treating FTO rs9939609 **AA**

DIET – first eight weeks

- Low fat, low sugar, higher protein. AA needs the highest amount of protein: 1 to 1.2 grams of protein per kilogram of body weight, divided by three, gives the amount of protein per meal. (For example, you weigh 80 kilograms. That's 80 to 96 grams of protein per day, allowing 27 to 32 grams per

meal.) Lower amounts of protein will increase food cravings and impair weight loss.
- Low saturated fat. Keep it to less than 30 grams per day.
    - *If your APOA2 coding is homozygous variant (CC), keep saturated fat to less than 22 grams of per day or 28 grams per day for heterozygous (CT).*
- Low sugar. Try to keep the majority of carbohydrates as vegetables and salads. These can be eaten in unlimited quantities. If you do wish to include grains, starches, fruits, sweets or alcohol, they can only be consumed at one meal per day and a portion size that is *at most* half the physical size of the protein.
    - *If your TCF7L2 coding is variant (CT) or (TT), reduce this portion size further to 1/3 the size of the protein.*
    - *If your IRS coding is variant (CC) or (CT), reduce this portion size further to 1/3 the size of the protein.*
- Consider intermittent fasting (I.F.). AA genotypes overall need fewer calories per day as they burn through them more slowly. They will see increased adiponectin levels and weight loss with an I.F. program. This incorporates two meals per day with one small snack in between if needed, all consumed within an eight-hour period, leaving the other 16 hours as fasting. During fasting, you can have fluids including coffee and tea (which can contain a small amount of milk but no sugar) and water. Avoid sugary drinks and fruit juice.
- *If you are an AA who does not need to lose weight, it is key to still keep the gene in check by following the dietary protocol above for the eight-week genetic retraining period. After the eight-week period, you can increase the healthy grains or starches or fruits to one per meal, but still keep the size to ½ the size of the protein. The FTO A-allele exerts a powerful influence, and even if you don't feel its effects now, factors such as stress and aging can turn it "on" in the future. Following this protocol will ensure this gene remains in its "off" position.*

> **Dietary Fats (see also Chapter 19 and Appendix 1 Food Tables)**
> - *Saturated fats are highest in fatty meats including lamb, beef and pork, processed meats such as bacon and sausage, full-fat dairy products, coconut and palm oil, cakes and pastries. Here are some examples:*
>
> | Food Source | Total Fat | Saturated Fat |
> |---|---|---|
> | 1 Whole Egg | 5 grams | 1.6 grams |
> | Beef 100g/3.5oz | 15 grams | 6 grams |
> | Lamb Chop 100g/3.5oz | 21 grams | 9 grams |
> | Bacon 100g/3.5oz | 42 grams | 14 grams |
> | Pork Sausage 100g/3.5oz | 20 grams | 7 grams |
> | Croissant 1 | 14 grams | 9 grams |
> | Whole Milk 1 cup | 8 grams | 5 grams |
> | Cheddar Cheese 2tbsp/30g | 8 grams | 6 grams |
> | Goat Cheese 2tbsp/30g | 9 grams | 6 grams |
> | Butter 1tbsp/15g | 12 grams | 7.3 grams |
> | Coconut Oil 1tbsp/15g | 14 grams | 13 grams |
> | 70% Dark Chocolate 2 squares/20g | 10 grams | 6 grams |
>
> - *Polyunsaturated fats are found in fatty fish such as salmon, mackerel, herring, flax seed and walnuts*
> - *Monounsaturated fats are found in avocados, olives, canola oil, almonds and walnuts*

DIET – after eight weeks

- You may add in a simple carbohydrate at a second meal, but it needs to remain at ½ the physical size of your protein portion.

This is a very good example of why certain diets are only appropriate for certain individuals. An FTO A carrier following a high-fat diet such as Keto Diet or the Bulletproof Diet would be consuming way above their 30 grams per day limit of saturated fat. The Keto Diet, for example, would contain 80 to 125 grams of fat per day, which will stimulate ghrelin, lower adiponectin and increase the risk of leptin resistance. They will increase fat cell capacity and inflammation, leading to more insulin resistance and the likelihood metabolic syndrome. This is why it is so important to assess your genetic metabolism before starting a new diet.

EXERCISE

- Physical inactivity greatly increases risk of weight gain and metabolic syndrome in A-allele carriers.
- Exercise helps to boost PGC1-α, which is converted to irisin, browning white fat and increasing thermogenesis. Exercise will also help regulate blood sugar and increase adiponectin. AA individuals should try to exercise while fasting as they will boost their adiponectin to a much higher level and utilize adipose tissue rather than glucose or glycogen as a fuel source.

SUPPLEMENTS

- Tri-Metabolic Control (TMC) – inhibits ghrelin, increases adiponectin and regulates leptin. Take two capsules twice a day 30 minutes to one hour before lunch and dinner. This should be taken for a minimum of eight weeks. After eight weeks, this should be cycled in one week out of every four weeks to maintain healthy hormonal levels. (See TMC note at the end of this chapter.)
- If you do not need to lose weight, then simply start by using TMC on the one-week-in-four regimen to maintain healthy hormone levels.
- Whey Satisfied Protein Powder – Take one scoop in water or almond milk at two meals a day. Note that this provides 10 grams of your protein requirement and regulates ghrelin and leptin.

The following additional supplements can be used to help curb food cravings. They are not necessarily needed by all AAs.

- L-Glutamine – binds to sweet receptors on the tongue and inhibits sugar cravings. Put one scoop in water, swish in mouth for 30 seconds and swallow for immediate reduction in sugar cravings.
- L-tyrosine or Dopaplus – boosts dopamine and inhibits cravings for fatty foods. Take one to two capsules twice a day on an empty stomach (30 minutes or more before a meal or two hours or more after food).

Note on TMC:
If you carry the A-allele (AA or TA), "turning off" this gene can be difficult, especially if you have a history of typically poor dietary habits, high stress and limited exercise. If you fall into this category, then TMC becomes even more important during the first eight weeks of genetic retraining while changing your lifestyle. After that, I recommend AAs and TAs cycling TMC one week out of every four to six weeks. You can also use it during periods of extra stress or when you fall off your diet for a few days such as when on holiday.

Tri-Metabolic Control (TMC)

TMC is a combination of Piper betle, Dolichos biflorus and acetyl-L-carnitine (ALCAR). The effect of Piper betle and Dolichos biflorus was compared to a placebo in an eight-week randomized, double-blind controlled study on individuals with high BMI. All participants ate a standardized 2,000-calorie diet and maintained the same intensity and duration of exercise five times a week. Participants taking the supplement combination demonstrated a decrease in ghrelin of 20% and an increase in adiponectin of 17%. In addition to these hormonal changes, the supplemented group had significantly more weight loss.

ALCAR helps to regulate leptin. Studies in rats (Iossa, 2002) show the impact ALCAR has on leptin. Rats with diet-induced leptin resistance were fed 15 milligrams per litre of ALCAR in their water for one month. Diet and exercise were held constant. At the end of the month, leptin levels stabilized, and there was a significant reduction in leptin resistance. An increase in ATP production was also seen. If both adiponectin and leptin are balanced at the same time, then the effect is far more powerful (almost double the response) than when treating either hormone alone.

Gene Integration

There are many genes that influence health and metabolism, so when performing my analysis, I take into account an individual's coding for a number of other related SNPs. There are some well-documented interactions between certain SNPs, and using this information along with my clinical experience, I have determined that patients with certain genotypes respond differently dependent on their coding for these complementary SNPs. These algorithms, which I have termed "SNP integration," are one of the unique features of my protocols (and my GeneRx.ca platform), and I find they greatly increase the individual specificity and success of treatment.

ADIPOQ rs17366568 variant (AA) or heterozygous (GA)
MC4R rs17782313 variant (CC) or heterozygous (TC)
Continue TMC for 8 to 12 weeks and then cycle it one week out of every four to six weeks thereafter.

APOA2 coding is homozygous variant (CC) or heterozygote (CT)
Keep saturated fat to less than 22 grams per day rather than 30 grams per day.

Try to keep the majority of carbohydrates as veggies and salads. If including grains, starches, fruits, sweets or alcohol, choose only one of these per meal and limit it to a portion size that is at most half the physical size of the protein.

TCF7L2 coding is variant (CT) or (TT)
IRS1 coding is variant (CC) or (CT)
Reduce carbohydrate portion size to ⅓ tcn rather than ½.

Treating FTO rs9939609 *TA*

DIET – first eight weeks

- Low fat, low sugar, average protein. TA needs an average amount of protein at each meal: 0.8 to 1.0 grams of protein per kilogram of body weight divided by three. More than this can inflame the body, and less than this will decrease satiety and reduce the rate of weight loss.
- Lower saturated fat. You do not need it as low as AAs but still require less saturated fat than TTs so as not to increase the expression of the A-allele. Keep saturated fat to less than 28 to 30 grams per day.
  - *If your APOA2 coding is homozygous variant (CC), keep saturated fat to less than 22 grams per day, or 28 grams per day for heterozygous (CT).*
- Low sugar. Try to keep the majority of carbohydrates as vegetables and salads. These can be eaten in unlimited quantities. If you do wish to include grains, starches, fruits, sweets or alcohol, they can only be consumed at two meals per day and a portion size that is *at most* half the physical size of the protein.
  - *If your TCF7L2 coding is variant (CT) or (TT), reduce this portion size further to 1/3 the size of the protein.*
  - *If your IRS coding is variant (CC) or (CT), reduce this portion size further to 1/3 the size of the protein.*
- Consider intermittent fasting. TA genotypes still require fewer calories per day than TTs, as they burn through them more slowly. They will see increased adiponectin levels and weight loss with an I.F. program. This incorporates two meals per day with one small snack in between if needed, all consumed within an eight-hour period, leaving the other 16 hours as fasting. During fasting, you can have fluids including coffee and tea

(can contain a small amount of milk but no sugar) and water. Avoid sugary drinks and fruit juice.
- *If you are a TA who does not need to lose weight, it is key to still keep the gene in check by following the dietary protocol above for the eight-week genetic retraining period. After the eight-week period, you can increase the healthy grains or starches or fruits to one per meal, but still keep the size to ½ the size of the protein. Doing this will ensure this gene remains in its "off" position, reduce inflammation and, most of all, prepare your genes for the future and prevent full expression of this gene and subsequent weight gain.*

DIET – after eight weeks

- You may add in a simple carbohydrate at a third meal (unless continuing intermittent fasting), but it needs to remain at ½ the physical size of your protein portion.

EXERCISE

- Physical inactivity greatly increases risk of weight gain and metabolic syndrome in A-allele carriers.
- Exercise helps to boost PGC1-α, which is converted to irisin, browning white fat and increasing thermogenesis. Exercise will also help regulate blood sugar and increase adiponectin. TA individuals should try to exercise while fasting as they will boost their adiponectin to a much higher level and utilize adipose tissue rather than glucose or glycogen as a fuel source.

SUPPLEMENTS

- Tri-Metabolic Control (TMC) – inhibits ghrelin, increases adiponectin and regulates leptin. Take two capsules twice a day 30 minutes to one hour before lunch and dinner. This should be taken for a minimum of eight weeks. After the eight weeks, this should be cycled in one week out of every four weeks to maintain healthy hormonal levels.

- If you do not need to lose weight, then simply start by using TMC on the one-week-in-four cycle regimen to maintain healthy hormone levels.
- Whey Satisfied Protein Powder – Take one scoop in water or almond milk at two meals a day. Note that this provides 10 grams of your protein requirement and regulates ghrelin and leptin.

The following additional supplements can be used to help curb food cravings. They are not necessarily needed by all TAs.

- L-Glutamine – binds to sweet receptors on the tongue and inhibits sugar cravings. Put one scoop in water, swish in mouth for 30 seconds and swallow for immediate reduction in sugar cravings.
- L-tyrosine or Dopaplus – boosts dopamine and inhibits cravings for fatty foods. Take one to two capsules twice a day on an empty stomach (30 minutes or more before a meal or two hours or more after food).

TMC Note:
If you carry the A-allele (AA or TA), "turning off" this gene can be difficult, especially if you have a history of typically poor dietary habits, high stress and limited exercise. If you fall into that category, then TMC becomes even more important during the first eight weeks of genetic retraining while changing your lifestyle. After that, I recommend AAs and TAs cycling TMC one week out of every four to six weeks. You can also use it during periods of extra stress or when you fall off your diet for a few days such as when on holiday.

Treating FTO rs9939609 *TT*

DIET – first eight weeks

- Moderate fat, moderate sugar, low protein. TTs needs the lowest amount of protein at each meal: 0.6 to 0.8 grams of

protein per kilogram of body weight divided by three. More than this can inflame the body, and less than this will decrease satiety and reduce the rate of weight loss (if part of your program).
- Moderate saturated fat. TTs are not as sensitive to saturated fats but excessive consumption can still be unhealthy. Keep saturated fat to less than 30 to 35 grams per day.
  - *If your APOA2 coding is homozygous variant (CC), keep saturated fat to less than 22 grams per day, or 28 grams per day for heterozygous (CT).*
- Moderate sugar. Although less important for TTs, from an overall health perspective, try to keep the majority of carbohydrates as vegetables and salads. If including grains, starches, fruits, sweets or alcohol, choose only one of these per meal and with a portion size that is up to two-thirds the physical size of the protein at each meal.
  - *If your TCF7L2 coding is variant (CT) or (TT), reduce this portion size to ½ the size of the protein.*
  - *If your IRS1 coding is variant (CC) or (CT), reduce this portion size further to ½ the size of the protein.*
- Intermittent fasting is not recommended for TTs.
- *If you are a TT who does not need to lose weight, follow the above dietary protocol. If you do need to lose weight, then reference your other genes as this is likely where changes are needed.*

DIET – after eight weeks

- No significant change

EXERCISE

- Exercise helps to boost PGC1-α, which is converted to irisin, browning white fat and increasing thermogenesis. Exercise will also help regulate blood sugar and increase adiponectin. TTs are often not suitable for exercise on an empty stomach. This will be somewhat dependent on certain exercise-related genes such as LIPC, PPARGC1A and LPL (genes not included in this book).

SUPPLEMENTS

- TTs generally do not need any special supplementation.

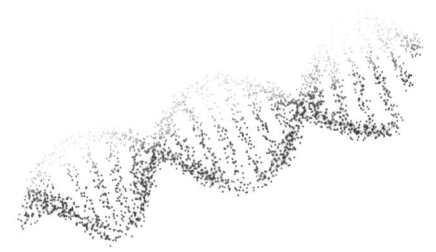

CHAPTER 9
ADIPOQ
The Adiponectin Fat Cell Messenger Gene

ADIPOQ Quick Look

ADIPOQ rs17366568 (weight loss)	ADIPOQ rs17300539 (weight maintenance)
<u>A-allele</u> (risk) • Lower circulating adiponectin during weight loss • Slower rate of weight loss • Increased overall weight gain and BMI • Unstable blood sugars, insulin levels • More food cravings • Food cravings disappear or lessen with calorie deprivation • Weight loss increases with calorie deprivation	<u>G-allele</u> (risk) • Regains weight easily after weight loss • Yo-yo dieter • More unstable glucose and insulin during weight maintenance • Increased weight and BMI • Increased food cravings during weight maintenance • Symptoms decrease with caloric restriction
<u>G-allele</u> (normal) • No risk; ideal coding	<u>A-allele</u> (normal) • No risk; ideal coding

The ADIPOQ gene codes for the 244-amino acid protein Adiponectin, circulating in high concentrations in the blood of normal individuals.

Adiponectin is a bioactive, fat cell–derived hormone (adipokine) produced primarily in adipose tissue. There is some production in bone marrow, the cardiovascular system, the liver and muscle mass, but it is produced in highest concentration in fatty tissue. It increases insulin sensitivity, at least partially, by suppressing glucose production, increases fatty acid oxidation and regulates glucose and insulin levels. It increases healthy fat storage while preventing accumulation of lipids in other tissues (liver, muscle and arteries, among others) and has a strong cardio-protective role. Adiponectin inhibits damaging inflammatory pathways, increasing endothelial nitrous oxide (NO) production and inhibiting oxidative stress. Adiponectin deficiency is associated with increased damage during cardiac ischemic events.

Reduced fat mass increases adiponectin, promoting glucose and fatty acid uptake into adipocytes. Adiponectin reduces the production of cholesterol and glucose by the liver so helps control metabolic syndrome. Overall, it has a profound effect on the storage and use of fat as an energy source, and extensive research indicates that it prevents the development of metabolic syndrome disorders such as diabetes. Circulating levels are significantly lower in patients with obesity, diabetes, hypertension and coronary artery disease, and research shows that adiponectin can reverse insulin resistance and may provide a novel treatment approach for type 2 diabetes.

Our genes can affect adiponectin level but so can our weight and adiposity. Clinically low levels are observed in obese or diabetic individuals. This may seem odd for a hormone that is made in the fat cells. One would think that more fat cells would mean more adiponectin production. But that is not the case. When weight starts to rise above normal, adiponectin levels begin to fall dramatically.

The paradox of a hormone that is produced by fat cells yet shows *decreased* levels in obesity is explained in part by the finding that adiponectin secretion by fat cells is *inversely* proportional to their size (diameter). In effect, obesity leads to dysfunctional fat cells that are no longer able to function effectively in controlling energy storage and metabolism. In contrast and possibly even more counterintuitive is that when calories are restricted and body mass falls, adiponectin levels begin to rise, an effect largely mediated by a switch to production by the fat cells in bone marrow.

Diet also has a profound effect on adiponectin production. High-saturated-fat intake increases blood sugar levels and decreases adiponectin, leading to insulin resistance, weight gain and impairment of fat burning in skeletal muscle. The same effect is not seen with polyunsaturated fats.

Stress has an ability to alter the expression of most genes. In fact, stress alters over 90% of genes, always increasing or decreasing their expression in an adverse way. Sadly, stress never directs our genes to make us sleep better, lose more weight or lower cholesterol. Excess glucocorticoids greatly *decrease* the production of adiponectin. To demonstrate this, scientists took a group of healthy patients and injected them with either 25 mg of hydrocortisone to mimic a stressful situation or a placebo (Fallo, 2004). Serum adiponectin levels were then measured at 1, 15, 30, 60, 120 and 180 minutes. When other variables were controlled for, they found that the hydrocortisone greatly reduced adiponectin levels in the healthy individuals at 30 and 60 minutes compared to the placebo group. They also found that adiponectin was significantly lower in non-obese Cushing's patients (patients with a disease that results in chronically high corticosteroid production) compared to the non-obese normal patients, indicating that glucocorticoids, from an endogenous or exogenous source, decrease the production of circulating adiponectin.

In another study (De Oliveira, 2011) looking at the combined effect of both diet and the stress hormone cortisol on adiponectin, rats were fed either a normal or high-fat diet for 12 weeks. As expected, the high-fat group demonstrated increased blood sugar levels and a fourfold reduction in ADIPOQ gene expression. The rats then underwent surgery to remove their adrenal glands to decrease their serum cortisol levels. Half the rats had the cortisol replaced with injections while the other half just got saline. The rats that had their cortisol replaced continued to show high levels of blood glucose and insulin along with reduced levels of circulating adiponectin. ADIPOQ gene expression in fat, liver and muscle tissue was up to seven times lower than normal. The rats that got saline and therefore on-going low cortisol normalized their glucose and insulin and increased their adipose tissue ADIPOQ expression fourfold. Persistent high-cortisol levels present in chronic stress can be expected to have a similar effect on adiponectin, glucose and insulin even with a relatively healthy diet.

As noted above, adiponectin has a strong cardio-protective role and inhibits damaging inflammatory pathways, increasing endothelial NO production and inhibiting oxidative stress. Low adiponectin levels are associated with cardiovascular disease. Experiments on human aortic endothelial cells show that adiponectin has a dose-dependent effect on the expression of tumour necrosis factor (TNF)–induced vascular cell adhesion molecules (VCAMs). VCAMs are proteins that promote the adherence of immune cells such as lymphocytes, monocytes and basophils to the inner lining of blood vessels, one of the earliest stages in atherosclerosis (Goldstein, 2009). These cardiovascular changes are also caused by high levels of circulating glucose, fat and insulin, which amplify the effects of low adiponectin.

There is ample evidence to support the association of certain ADIPOQ SNPs with vascular disease, including both clinical and subclinical cardiovascular disease, large vessel disease and intracranial vasculopathy. Study results can be difficult to interpret and extrapolate due to the large number of different ADIPOQ SNPs tested and the fact that risk varies considerably across different ethnic populations. However, the suggestion is that SNPs associated with low adiponectin likely have significant influence over a number of diseases, particularly those associated with metabolic syndrome and obesity.

Possibly as a result of increased inflammation, low levels of adiponectin are associated with an increased risk of certain obesity-related cancers such as colorectal and gastric cancer.

Treatment is aimed at increasing adiponectin levels, adjusting dietary intake to mitigate any effects of low adiponectin and reducing cortisol, which as we have seen, further impairs adiponectin production. Besides improving weight management, optimizing adiponectin has the potential to reduce long-term risk of insulin resistance and type 2 diabetes. It may also prove beneficial in terms of vascular disease and obesity-related cancers.

ADIPOQ SNPs

There are two main ADIPOQ SNPs:
- ADIPOQ rs17366568 codes for the production of adiponectin during weight loss
- ADIPOQ rs17300539 codes for the production of adiponectin during weight maintenance

ADIPOQ rs17366568
This codes for the production of adiponectin during **weight loss**.
Normal/Ancestral allele – G
Variant/Risk allele – A

A-allele:
- Lower circulating adiponectin during weight loss
- Slower rate of weight loss
- Increased overall weight gain and BMI
- Unstable blood sugars, insulin levels
- More food cravings
- Food cravings disappear or lessen with calorie deprivation
- Weight loss increases with calorie deprivation

During periods of weight loss, the A-allele is associated with lower circulating adiponectin levels compared to the G-allele. This makes losing weight much harder. There is instability of glucose and insulin levels and increased food cravings. Overall, metabolism and fat burning are slowed.

ADIPOQ rs17300539
This codes for the production of adiponectin during *weight maintenance*.
Normal/Ancestral allele – A
Variant/Risk allele – G

G-allele:
- Regains weight easily after weight loss
- Yo-yo dieter
- More unstable glucose and insulin during weight maintenance
- Increased weight and BMI
- Increased food cravings during weight maintenance
- Symptoms decrease with caloric restriction

During steady-state periods of weight maintenance, individuals with the G-allele have lower adiponectin production and thus an increased risk of unwanted weight gain. For those that struggle with dieting, the G-allele significantly increases the risk of regaining weight lost during a previous diet, often resulting in "yo-yo dieting."

TREATMENT - WEIGHT LOSS

ADIPOQ The Adiponectin Fat Cell Messenger Gene rs17366568 Weight Loss
Normal/Ancestral allele – G
Variant/Risk allele – A

Treating ADIPOQ rs17366568 **AA**
This SNP results in greatly lowered adiponectin production during weight loss.

DIET – first eight weeks
- Intermittent fasting. Two meals per day with one small snack in between if needed, all consumed within an eight-hour period, leaving the other 16 hours as fasting with just fluids such as coffee, tea (can have a small amount of milk in it but less than 20 calories) and water.

- Reduce calories to 800 to 1,000 per day.
- For other guidelines on protein, carbohydrate and fat, please refer to your other genes (FTO, TCF7L2, IRS1, APOA2 and FABP2).

DIET – after 8 weeks

- You can move to three meals a day (with *no snacks*) if you wish, but continuing I.F. would be ideal for this coding.

EXERCISE

- No specific exercise guidelines relating to ADIPOQ

SUPPLEMENTS

- Tri-Metabolic Control (TMC) – inhibits ghrelin, increases adiponectin and regulates leptin
- TMC for eight weeks. Take two capsules twice a day 30 minutes to one hour before lunch and dinner. If intermittent fasting (two meals only per day) and choosing breakfast and lunch, adjust according to your meal timing.
- After eight weeks:
    - If normal (AA) for ADIPOQ rs17300539 (see below), stop TMC.
    - If variant (GG) or heterozygous (AG) for ADIPOQ rs17300539 (see below), then cycle TMC (two capsules twice a day) one week out of every four to six weeks to prevent adiponectin from falling again.
    - If you are variant (AA) or heterozygote (TA) for FTO (see previous chapter), then cycle TMC (two capsules twice a day) one week out of every four to six weeks.
- In the event of significant deviation from your genetic diet (including snacking and "cheating" for three or more consecutive days) or if on a holiday, for example, where your diet may be compromised, then take TMC (two capsules twice a day) during the event or for three or four days afterward.

Treating ADIPOQ rs17366568 **GA**
This SNP results in lowered adiponectin production during weight loss.

DIET – first eight weeks

- Intermittent fasting. Two meals per day with one small snack in between if needed, all consumed within an eight-hour period, leaving the other 16 hours as fasting with just fluids such as coffee, tea (can have a small amount of milk in it but less than 20 calories) and water.
- Reduce calories to 900 to 1,200 per day.
- For other guidelines on protein, carbohydrate and fat, please refer to your other genes (FTO, TCF7L2, IRS1, APOA2 and FABP2).

DIET – after 8 weeks

- You can move to three meals a day (with *no snacks*) if you wish, but continuing I.F. would be ideal for this coding.

EXERCISE

- No specific exercise guidelines relating to ADIPOQ

SUPPLEMENTS

- TMC for six weeks. Take two capsules twice a day 30 minutes to one hour before lunch and dinner. If intermittent fasting (two meals only per day) and choosing breakfast and lunch, adjust according to your meal timing.
- After six weeks:
  - If normal (AA) for ADIPOQ rs17300539 (see below), stop TMC.
  - If variant (GG) or heterozygous (AG) for ADIPOQ rs17300539 (see below), then cycle TMC (two capsules twice a day) one week out of every four to six weeks to prevent adiponectin from falling again.

- If you are variant (AA) or heterozygote (TA) for FTO (see previous chapter), then cycle TMC (two capsules twice a day) one week out of every four to six weeks.
- In the event of significant deviation from your genetic diet (including snacking and "cheating" for three or more consecutive days) or if on a holiday, for example, where your diet may be compromised, then take TMC (two capsules twice a day) during the event or for three or four days afterward.

Treating ADIPOQ rs17366568 **GG**

This SNP results in normal adiponectin production during weight loss.

- Follow a genetic diet according to your FTO, TCF7L2, IRS1, APOA2 and FABP22 genes

TREATMENT - WEIGHT MAINTENANCE

ADIPOQ The Adiponectin Fat Cell Messenger Gene rs17300539 Weight Maintenance

Normal/Ancestral allele – A
Variant/Risk allele – G

I recommend you start treating this SNP once you have completed the eight-week retraining program for your other genes. Note that I would generally not include specific treatment recommendations for this SNP in someone with no weight issues. However, instituting the protocol below may confer some benefit in terms of increasing levels of adiponectin and reducing vascular inflammation.

Treating ADIPOQ rs17300539 **GG**

This SNP results in greatly lowered adiponectin production during **weight maintenance**.

DIET

- Intermittent fasting. Two meals per day with one small snack in between if needed, all consumed within an eight-hour period, leaving the other 16 hours as fasting with just fluids such as coffee, tea (can have a small amount of milk in it but less than 20 calories) and water.
- Reduce calories to 800 to 1,000 per day.
- For other guidelines on protein, carbohydrate and fat, please refer to your other genes (FTO, TCF7L2, IRS1, APOA2 and FABP2).

EXERCISE

- No specific exercise guidelines relating to ADIPOQ

SUPPLEMENTS

- TMC. Take two capsules twice a day 30 minutes to one hour before lunch and dinner one week in every four to six weeks. If intermittent fasting (two meals only per day) and choosing breakfast and lunch, adjust according to your meal timing.
- If you are variant (AA) or heterozygote (TA) for FTO (see previous chapter), then cycle TMC (two capsules twice a day) one week out of every two to three weeks.
- In the event of significant deviation from your genetic diet (including snacking and "cheating" for three or more consecutive days) or if on a holiday, for example, where your diet may be compromised, then take TMC (two capsules twice a day) during the event or for three or four days afterward.

Treating ADIPOQ rs17300539 AG
This SNP results in lowered adiponectin production during **weight maintenance**.

DIET

- Intermittent fasting. Two meals per day with one small snack in between if needed, all consumed within an eight-hour period, leaving the other 16 hours as fasting with just fluids such as coffee, tea (can have a small amount of milk in it but less than 20 calories) and water.
- Reduce calories to 900 to 1,200 per day.
- For other guidelines on protein, carbohydrate and fat, please refer to your other genes (FTO, TCF7L2, IRS1, APOA2 and FABP2).

EXERCISE

- No specific exercise guidelines relating to ADIPOQ

SUPPLEMENTS

- TMC. Take two capsules twice a day 30 minutes to one hour before lunch and dinner one week every five to seven weeks. If intermittent fasting (two meals only per day) and choosing breakfast and lunch, adjust dosing according to your meal timing.
- If you are variant (AA) or heterozygote (TA) for FTO (see previous chapter), then cycle TMC (two capsules twice a day) one week out of every two to three weeks.
- In the event of significant deviation from your genetic diet (including snacking and "cheating" for three or more consecutive days) or if on a holiday, for example, where your diet may be compromised, then take TMC (two capsules twice a day) during the event or for three or four days afterward.

Treating ADIPOQ rs17300539 ***AA***
This SNP results in normal adiponectin production during **weight loss**.

- Follow your genetic diet according to your other genes

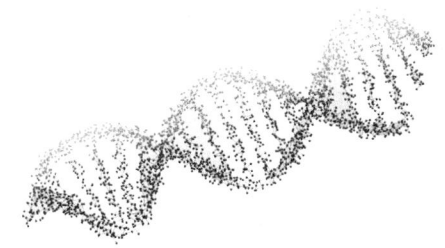

CHAPTER 10

MC4R

The Melanocortin-4 Receptor Satiety Gene
rs17782313
Normal/Ancestral allele – T
Variant/Risk allele – C

MC4R Quick Look

MC4R C-allele (risk)
- One C-allele is associated with an 8% increase in obesity. Each C-allele increases BMI by 0.22 units
- The homozygote variant CC can increase body weight by up to 43% independent of diet and exercise and increase BMI by 0.44 units
- Decreased satiety, increased appetite and snacking, especially with foods high in saturated fat
- Strong association with emotional and stress-related overeating
- Weight gain on antidepressants and antipsychotics
- Increased insulin resistance and a 14% increase in risk for type 2 diabetes

MC4R T-allele (normal)
- No risk; ideal coding

The MC4R gene codes for the Melanocortin-4 receptor. These receptors are located predominantly in the hypothalamus of the brain. where they play a central role in satiety and the control of food intake. When stimulated by the agonist neuropeptide α-MSH (alpha melanocyte stimulating hormone), they reduce hunger, improve sensitivity to satiety signals, promote meal termination and increase metabolism, fat burning and thermogenesis. Therefore, the MC4 receptor plays a pivotal role in the tonic control of food intake, energy expenditure and weight homeostasis.

Mutations in the structure of the MC4 receptor have a profound impact on hunger, food intake, energy metabolism and adiposity. Animals with MC4 receptor mutations show hyperphagia (excess eating), delayed meal termination and reduced sensitivity to satiety feedback peptides such as CCK (cholecystokinin). They also demonstrate metabolic abnormalities including reduced insulin sensitivity, impaired thermogenesis and lowered overall metabolic rate. Similar findings are seen in humans. A number of mutations with varying effect and penetrance (influence) are associated with obesity and metabolic syndrome. Individuals with genetic variance in MC4R (often called MC4R deficiency) tend to gain weight from early childhood, increasing both lean mass and adiposity. Such increased linear growth may in part be mediated by disproportionate early hyperinsulinemia.

The melanocortin system is interesting in that it is one of the few neuroendocrine systems that has a natural antagonist, in this case AgRP (agouti-related peptide). This messenger binds to the MC4 receptor and turns it off, which results in hunger, food-seeking behaviour, lowered metabolism and weight gain. Overexpression of the AgRP gene leads to obesity in mice, and there is evidence that certain SNPs in humans, which *lower* AgRP expression, are associated with resistance to weight gain (see Figure 1, page 92).

Neuropeptides controlling hunger and satiety have their effects mediated by the melanocortin system. Leptin, our "satiety hormone," exerts its hunger-suppressing effect by increasing α-MSH production and decreasing AgRP production. This leads to increased MC4R stimulation, reduced food intake and higher metabolism. Leptin resistance results in impairment of this effect and poor satiety signalling.

Hunger is stimulated in the brain by NPY (neuropeptide Y) acting on the sympathetic system and by AgRP inhibiting the MC4 receptors. Ghrelin, our "hunger hormone," acts to increase NPY and AgRP expression, resulting in food-seeking behaviour.

With such a central role in the overall control of hunger, food intake and metabolism, it is easy to see how subtle changes in the MC4 receptor can have a profound effect on weight homeostasis.

MC4R SNP rs17782313
Normal/Ancestral allele – T
Variant/Risk allele – C

Variations in the MC4R gene represent the most common form of monogenic obesity. A defect or variance in this gene results in fewer MC4 receptors and thus decreased function. When there are not enough receptors available, the "stop-eating" signal is impaired, and individuals never get the message to stop seeking out food. As the melanocortin system and MC4 receptors act as a tonic control over the drive to eat, even a small reduction in function or activity results in unchecked activity in the "hunger centre." The subsequent message the body receives is that it does not have enough energy stores and that for survival it needs to keep eating. This drive leads to increased food-seeking behaviour, impaired post-meal satiety and, thus, overeating. MC4R interacts extensively with the serotonin and dopamine pathways of the brain and therefore has an influence on both mood and reward. Studies have shown that individuals with the C-allele genotype have a significantly increased risk of depressed mood, and emotional eating is associated with the C-allele individual rather than the T-allele.

Dopamine activity is vital for proper functioning of the brain's reward pathways. This explains why under-expression of the dopamine DRD2 receptor is associated with reward deficiency syndrome and addiction. Such disorders include food addiction, which results in overeating and binge eating. Research indicates that MC4R and DRD2 work synergistically to control energy homeostasis and to integrate food reward and eating behaviour. In rats, administration of the MC4R antagonist AgRP activates dopaminergic neurons in the midbrain reward centres and promotes ingestion of highly palatable fat-rich foods. The melanocortin system and MC4 receptor therefore appear to have a dual role in controlling food intake. MC4R activity promotes satiety and reduces hunger as well as modulating the reward system to make food less attractive. This close interaction likely accounts for the effect the MC4R variant (C) allele has on cravings and mood-associated food intake.

The importance of stress in the expression of variant genotypes is not to be underestimated. In one study (Park, 2016) looking at the association of the variant MC4R C-allele with obesity, once adjusted for other variables, the results indicated that those individuals with high stress levels had a stronger association with higher BMI and preferential intake of processed and fat-dense foods over fruits and vegetables. The authors concluded that the interaction of stress and the variant allele of MC4R altered energy intake and eating behaviour to an extent that exceeded that of the variant allele alone. This represents a typical example of the epigenetic influence of stress. Leptin and insulin act in the brain to reduce appetite and food intake through activation of POMC neurons and the suppression of the MC4R antagonist AgRP. Individuals with the variant C-allele have resistance to the cerebral effects of insulin and leptin, which reduces their ability to achieve feedback suppression of appetite. This, combined with an overall higher level of blood sugar, increases the risk of type 2 diabetes.

Interestingly, individuals with reduced MC4R activity have a lower risk of high blood pressure. Research studies show that an intact MC4R system is required to induce the sympathetic nervous system stimulation required for hypertension. However, there appear to be other pathways by which adiposity increases blood pressure such that the MC4R variant allele does not provide comprehensive protection against this cardiovascular risk.

Effects of the MC4R C-allele
- One C-allele is associated with an 8% increase in obesity. And in fact, this mutation is the most common single genetic cause of obesity known to date (42% of the population has it [*SNPedia*]). Each C-allele increases BMI by 0.22 units.
- The homozygote variant CC can increase body weight by up to 43% independent of diet and exercise and increases BMI by 0.44 units.
- The C-allele results in decreased levels of satiety, causing more frequent eating and snacking, especially with foods high in saturated fat.
- The C-allele has a strong association with emotional overeating and is linked to an increased risk of depression.
- Individuals with the C-allele demonstrate greater stress-related cravings for processed foods.
- C-allele carriers experience rapid weight gain on antidepressants and antipsychotics.
- The C-allele is associated with increased insulin resistance and a 14% increase in risk for type 2 diabetes.

TREATMENT
MC4R The Melanocortin-4 Gene rs17782313
Normal/Ancestral allele – T
Variant/Risk allele – C

Treating MC4R rs17782313 **CC**

CC individuals benefit greatly from reduced food intake for both weight loss and weight maintenance. The overall amount (calories) of food should be limited and meal frequency reduced. *Unlike other metabolic SNPs, treatment for MC4R is long term with no initial eight-week retraining period.*

- Low-calorie diet – 800 to 1,100 calories per day dependent on your size, activity level and response
- Intermittent fasting. This incorporates two meals per day with one small snack in between if needed, all consumed within an eight-hour period, leaving the other 16 hours as fasting. During fasting, you can have fluids including coffee and tea (which can contain a small amount of milk but no sugar) and water. Avoid sugary drinks and fruit juice.
- In terms of protein, carbohydrate and fat, follow the guidelines according to your other genes (FTO, TCF7L2, IRS1, APOA2 and FABP2) but ensure you maintain the calorie and intermittent fasting rules.
- *If you are a CC who does not need to lose weight, I recommend following the intermittent fasting regimen but with slightly higher caloric intake (likely closer to the 1,100-calorie-per-day guideline).*
- As noted above. For this SNP coding, you should make this dietary regimen your normal routine.

EXERCISE

- No specific exercise guidelines relating to MC4R. However, increasing your overall activity level may allow a higher calorie intake and will help control cravings by increasing dopamine and serotonin levels.

SUPPLEMENTS

- Tri-Metabolic Control (TMC) – inhibits ghrelin, increases adiponectin and regulates leptin. Take two capsules twice a day 30 minutes to one hour before lunch and dinner. This should be taken for a minimum of eight weeks. After the eight weeks, this should be cycled, one week on and one week off to maintain healthy hormonal levels.

- Whey Satisfied Protein Powder. Put one scoop in water or almond milk at two meals a day. Note that this provides 10 grams of your protein requirement and regulates ghrelin and leptin.

For CC individuals, the priority is diet, TMC and Whey Satisfied Protein Powder.

Additional supplements, if needed:

- If you are prone to unstable blood sugar (light-headed or dizzy, anxious or "hangry," or feel hungry quickly):
    - Metabolic Xtra. Take one capsule twice a day on an empty stomach.
- If you are prone to food cravings:
    - DopaPlus (FocusPlus in Canada) or L-Tyrosine. Take one or two capsules twice a day on an empty stomach (30 minutes before food or at least two hours after). This can also be taken on an "as-needed" basis at times of craving.
    - L-Glutamine. Take one scoop dissolved in water or one capsule as needed for sweet craving.

Treating MC4R rs17782313 **TC**

Due to the significant influence of the C-allele, TC treatment is the same as for CC. Individuals benefit greatly from reduced food intake for both weight loss and weight maintenance. The overall amount (calories) of food should be limited and meal frequency reduced. *Unlike other metabolic SNPs, treatment for MC4R is long term with no initial eight-week retraining period.*

- Low-calorie diet. Eat 800 to 1,100 calories per day dependent on your size, activity level and response.

- Intermittent fasting. This incorporates two meals per day with one small snack in between if needed, all consumed within an eight-hour period, leaving the other 16 hours as fasting. During fasting, you can have fluids including coffee and tea (which can contain a small amount of milk but no sugar) and water. Avoid sugary drinks and fruit juice.
- In terms of protein, carbohydrate and fat, follow the guidelines according to your other genes (FTO, TCF7L2, IRS1, APOA2 and FABP2) but ensure you maintain the calorie and intermittent fasting rules.
- *If you are a TC who does not need to lose weight, I recommend following the intermittent fasting regimen but with slightly higher caloric intake (likely closer to the 1,100-calorie-per-day guideline).*
- *As noted above. For this SNP coding, you should make this dietary regimen your normal routine.*

EXERCISE

- No specific exercise guidelines relating to MC4R. However, increasing your overall activity level may allow a higher calorie intake and will help control cravings by increasing dopamine and serotonin levels.

SUPPLEMENTS

- Tri-Metabolic Control (TMC) – inhibits ghrelin, increases adiponectin and regulates leptin. Take two capsules twice a day 30 minutes to one hour before lunch and dinner. This should be taken for a minimum of eight weeks. After the eight weeks, this should be cycled, one week on and one week off to maintain healthy hormonal levels.
- Whey Satisfied Protein Powder. Take one scoop in water or almond milk at two meals a day. Note that this provides 10 grams of your protein requirement and regulates ghrelin and leptin.

For TC individuals, the priority is diet, TMC and Whey Satisfied Protein Powder.

Additional supplements, if needed:

- If you are prone to unstable blood sugar (light-headed or dizzy, anxious or "hangry," or feel hungry quickly):
  - Metabolic Xtra. Take one capsule twice a day on an empty stomach.
- If you are prone to food cravings:
  - DopaPlus (FocusPlus in Canada) or L-Tyrosine. Take one or two capsules twice a day on an empty stomach (30 minutes before food or at least two hours after). This can also be taken on an "as-needed" basis at times of craving.
  - L-Glutamine. Take one scoop dissolved in water or one capsule as needed for sweet craving.

Treating MC4R rs17782313 TT

TT is the optimal coding and poses no additional risks.

- Follow your genetic diet according to your other genes

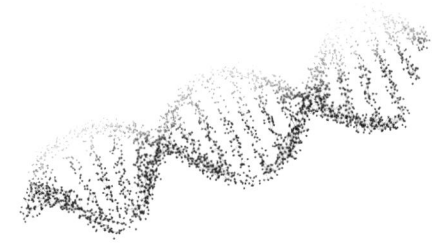

CHAPTER 11
PPARG

The Fatty Acid and Glucose Metabolism Gene
rs1801282
Normal/Ancestral allele – C
Variant allele – G

PPARG Quick Look

G-allele – this is the variant allele but is healthier
- *Lower BMI*
- *Improved insulin sensitivity*
- *Reduced risk of type 2 diabetes*
- *Lower heart disease risk*
- *Worse on a high-saturated-fat and high-carbohydrate diet*
- *Higher BMI on a diet with high saturated-to-polyunsaturated fat ratio*
- *Significant cumulative effect when it interacts with other polymorphisms especially FTO, LEPR, ADIPOQ, MC4R and ADRA*
- *Good weight-loss response with caloric reduction*
- *Improved health benefits from exercise*
- **Higher risk of complications in patients that develop diabetes**
- **Increased weight gain if the individual becomes overweight**

> **Note**: PPARG is one of those unusual SNPs for which the variant or risk allele (G) actually confers health benefits rather than being detrimental. The caveat to this is that should individuals with the G-allele become overweight, their risk for additional weight gain is increased. In addition, even though the SNP reduces the likelihood of diabetes, should someone with the G-allele actually become diabetic, their risk for developing the complications associated with this disorder is much higher.
>
> **C-allele** – this is the normal allele but imposes risk
> - Higher BMI
> - Reduced insulin sensitivity
> - Increased risk of type 2 diabetes
> - Worse on a high-carbohydrate and high-saturated-fat diet
> - Significant cumulative effect when it interacts with other polymorphisms especially FTO, TCF7L2, MC4R and APOA2
> - Improved blood sugar stability with caloric reduction
> - Fewer health benefits from exercise compared to GG

PPARG is a complex gene working through numerous mechanisms. It has an important role in glucose and fat metabolism, insulin sensitivity and inflammation.

Peroxisome Proliferator-Activated Receptor Gamma (PPAR-gamma, PPARG, Pro12Ala) or the glitazone receptor is a type-1 nuclear receptor (NR1C3) encoded by the PPARG gene. It plays a central role in fatty acid and glucose metabolism as well as fat storage and insulin sensitivity. It is found mostly in adipose tissue but is also seen in the lining of blood vessels and the colon and in macrophages. The receptor is the target for the TZD (thiazolidinediones) class of diabetic medications, which work by stimulating the PPARG receptor to increase adipogenesis and fatty acid uptake by peripheral tissues. The resulting decrease in fatty acid availability improves insulin sensitivity. The gene product has several different functions and has been coined the master regulator of adipocyte biology. It works by modifying the transcription of a number of genes involved in glucose and lipid metabolism, fat cell differentiation and energy balance. It also has an anti-inflammatory effect on the endothelial cells of the cardiovascular system and reduces the development of atherosclerosis. Its effect on inflammation may be even more widespread, with some studies indicating an association with conditions such as rheumatoid arthritis.

PPARG inhibits the expression of inflammatory cytokines such as TNF-a and IL-6, and directs the differentiation of immune cells toward anti-inflammatory phenotypes. Both synthetic and natural PPARG activators are currently under investigation for their potential as anti-inflammatory agents.

PPARG is shown to be an important factor in fat-cell differentiation. This process of adipogenesis involves the development of adipocyte precursor cells into functioning fat cells capable of filling with lipids and expressing adipokines such as leptin and adiponectin. PPARG has also been shown to promote the browning of white fat, a beneficial process that increases metabolism and fat burning and combats obesity. PPARG also appears to reduce the expression of resistin, an adipokine produced by adipocytes known to cause insulin resistance.

PPARG has an anti-cancer effect, controlling genes involved in cellular differentiation and regulating the cell cycle. It induces the tumour-suppressor gene PTEN and directly inhibits the proliferation of malignant cells from many cancer types including bladder, gastric, colorectal, breast, prostate, lung and brain.

PPAR is one of the genes exhibiting diurnal variation in expression and is an integral part of the circadian rhythm controlling energy metabolism and fat storage. Interestingly, it is also involved in bone metabolism.

The genetic mechanisms through which PPAR acts and its numerous isoforms (PPARA, PPARD, PPARG) contribute to significant confusion and controversy when it comes to its beneficial and potentially harmful effects. However, the weight of research indicates that it improves insulin sensitivity and protects against type 2 diabetes and metabolic syndrome.

PPAR-gamma SNP rs1801282
(Also called PPAR-gamma, PPARG and Pro12Ala polymorphism)
Normal/Ancestral allele – C (encodes for Pro sequence)
Variant/Risk allele – G (encodes for Ala sequence)

PPARG is one of those unusual SNPs for which the variant or risk allele (G) actually confers *health benefits* rather than being detrimental. The caveat is that should individuals with the G-allele become overweight, their risk for additional weight gain is increased. In addition, even though the SNP reduces the likelihood of diabetes, should someone with the G-allele actually become diabetic, their risk for developing the complications associated with this disorder is much higher.

G-allele
- Lower BMI
- Improved insulin sensitivity
- Reduced risk of type 2 diabetes
- Lower heart disease risk
- Worse on a high-saturated-fat and high-carbohydrate diet
- Higher BMI on a diet with high saturated-to-polyunsaturated fat ratio
- Significant cumulative effect when combined with other polymorphisms especially FTO, LEPR, ADIPOQ, MC4R and ADRA
- Good weight-loss response with caloric reduction
- Improved health benefits from exercise
- **Higher risk of complications in patients that develop diabetes**
- **Increased weight gain if the individual becomes overweight**

The G-allele is the variant allele and has a lower frequency within the population. Homozygous G-allele frequencies are 12% in Caucasians,

10% in Native Americans, 8% in Samoans, 4% in Japanese, 3% in African-Americans and 1% in Chinese. Caucasians have the highest G-allele frequency (GG and CG), resulting in a carrier prevalence of nearly 25%.

As opposed to many SNPs, it is the **normal** allele that appears to confer significant health risk. The individual effect may be quite small, but the population risk is high due to the prevalence of the C-allele (80 to 90%).

The C-allele is associated with:
- Higher BMI
- Reduced insulin sensitivity
- Increased risk of type 2 diabetes
- Worse on a high-carbohydrate and high-saturated-fat diet
- Significant cumulative effect when combines with other polymorphisms especially FTO, TCF7L2, MC4R and APOA2
- Improved blood sugar stability with caloric reduction

On the other hand, the variant G-allele is the one that confers a health benefit. The reason for this is not known, but it may represent an evolutionary attempt at protective adaptation to our modern dietary excess. Unfortunately, the allele is not infallible, and although it provides initial protection against obesity and diabetes, persistently poor diet will negate its positive effects.

The precise effect of the variant G-allele remains a subject of much discussion as its frequency varies greatly across ethnic populations, and its association with diabetes risk, metabolic syndrome, insulin resistance, weight gain and hyperlipidemia is often confusing in the scientific literature. However, the G-allele certainly appears to be associated with improved insulin sensitivity and a **reduced** risk of developing type 2 diabetes *in normal weight individuals*. Its frequency in the diabetic population is significantly lower than in those with normal glucose control. In one study, only 2.2% of subjects with diabetes had the variant SNP while 9.3% of the normal subjects exhibited it.

Another way of explaining this is to say that if the entire population carried the G-allele, then the prevalence of type 2 diabetes would be 25% lower. The harmful adipokine resistin is known to induce insulin resistance and increase the risk of type 2 diabetes. The G-allele is associated with **lower** levels of resistin, which is beneficial, while the C-allele **increases** resistin, particularly when combined with the GG phenotype of the resistin SNP rs1862513.

There is some evidence to indicate that G-allele carriers have increased BMI on the basis that lipolysis is impaired and fatty acid storage increased as a result of increased insulin sensitivity. This may account for some research showing the G-allele to be associated with increased serum cholesterol and triglycerides. The G-allele also predisposes to a higher BMI in carriers that consume a diet high in polyunsaturated fats. This is an example of a gene–diet interaction.

The fact that expression of this gene is both highly sensitive to dietary content and to the effects of other gene polymorphisms likely accounts for much of the variability in BMI association seen across different populations. What is quite clear, however, is that individuals with the G-allele that do end up developing type 2 diabetes seem to have a more profound effect of the disease including more rapid deterioration of pancreatic beta-cell function, higher levels of HbA1c, increased weight gain, higher serum cholesterol and triglycerides, higher BMI and increased blood pressure. They also have increased risk of diabetes-related inflammatory pathology such as atherosclerosis and heart disease.

On the plus side, those with the G-allele experience much greater improvements in glucose and insulin metabolism in response to regular endurance training than those with the C-allele.

But if PPARG increases insulin sensitivity, then why does the reduction in transcription associated with the G-allele result in *improved* sensitivity and a reduced risk of type 2 diabetes? One theory is that reduced PPAR transcription in adipocytes actually enhances the effect of insulin, decreasing lipolysis and FFA release. This would increase muscle utilization of glucose and reduce glucose production by the liver, thereby improving glucose control. The G-allele also results in a decrease in TNF-alpha and resistin production by adipocytes and an increase in adiponectin. These modulations will both increase insulin sensitivity. This theory is supported by the finding of increased PPARG expression in the adipocytes of obese individuals when compared to those of normal weight individuals. A calorie-restricted diet downregulates (reduces) PPARG expression and is therefore an important part of the treatment protocol.

Thus, having the G-allele would initially appear to be highly beneficial. However, in an environment where food is readily available and fats are a significant part of our diet, the G-allele may end up being detrimental. While the allele provides initial protection against obesity and diabetes, a persistently poor diet will eventually lead to increased adiposity, and this seems to reverse the effects of the allele. In fact, once BMI increases, the risk of further weight gain and the development of diabetes go up. Once an individual becomes diabetic, then the G-allele confers an increased risk of diabetic complications. This nutrigenetic or epigenetic influence on a gene likely represents a significant etiological contribution to diabetes and metabolic syndrome. Although evidence points to a role for genetic polymorphisms in the development of this epidemic disease, there is equally good research to support significant environmental causation.

The G-allele also confers an anti-inflammatory benefit, and its effect on lipid metabolism and insulin sensitivity is, at least in part, the result of reduced adipose tissue inflammation. This may also explain why the G-allele is protective against atherosclerosis and symptomatic coronary artery disease causing disability or death. One study found that each copy of the G-allele reduced ischemic heart disease risk by 90% and vascular death by 76% (Regieli, 2009).

TREATMENT

PPAR-gamma The Fatty Acid and Glucose Metabolism Gene rs1801282

Normal/Ancestral allele – C (**Risk allele**)
Variant allele – G (**Healthier allele**)

Treating PPAR-gamma rs1801282 **GG**

The homozygous variant coding of GG is ideal for this SNP and confers a health benefit rather than a risk. However, treatment for normal weight GG individuals aims to prevent weight gain and the development of diabetes as this allele is associated with increased adiposity and a higher risk of complications if either of these situations occur. If already overweight, then treatment for GG individuals involves a more aggressive weight loss regimen to take them out of the risk category for this genotype.

DIET FOR NORMAL-WEIGHT INDIVIDUALS – first eight weeks

- Moderate caloric intake – 1,000 to 1,200 calories per day
- Lower simple carbohydrate intake (see Chapter 19 for more information)
- Maintain a higher ratio of poly- or monounsaturated fat to saturated fat in the diet
- Keep saturated fat to a maximum of 30 grams per day
- If you are CC for APOA2 or AA for FTO, further reduce saturated fat to 22 grams per day
- Intermittent fasting not recommended (poorly tolerated)

DIET FOR OVERWEIGHT INDIVIDUALS – first eight weeks

- Low caloric intake – 900 to 1,000 calories per day
- Very low simple carbohydrate intake
- Maintain a higher ratio of poly- or monounsaturated fat to saturated fat in the diet

- Keep saturated fat to a maximum of 26 grams per day
- If you are CC for APOA2 or AA for FTO, further reduce saturated fat to 22 grams per day

DIET – after 8 weeks

- For this coding, I recommend you maintain the same dietary guidelines after the eight-week retraining period but you can increase your calorie intake to 1,200 calories per day if you wish.

FATS *(also see Appendix 1 Food Tables)*
- *Saturated fats = beef, pork, sausage, processed meats such as salami, chicken, butter, cheese, dairy products, coconut oil, MCT oil*

  Here are some examples of saturated fat levels (g = grams; oz = ounces; tbsp = tablespoons). Note: 1 oz = 28.35 g. Food amounts are given in ounces as this is the more typical measure in North America.
  - *coconut oil – 16 g/oz*
  - *butter – 7.6 g/tbsp*
  - *dark chocolate – 9.4 g/oz*
  - *hard goat cheese – 7 g/oz*
  - *almonds (approximately 30 almonds) – 1.1 g/oz*
  - *walnuts – 3 g in 12 walnuts*
  - *salmon – 6 g/7 oz (half a fillet)*
  - *beef – 13 g/3 oz (typical minimum beef serving in American restaurants is 8 oz)*
- *Polyunsaturated fats = fatty fish such as salmon, mackerel, herring, flax seed and walnuts*
- *Monounsaturated fats = avocados, olives, canola oil, almonds, walnuts*

EXERCISE FOR NORMAL AND OVERWEIGHT INDIVIDUALS

- GG variants show improved glucose and insulin metabolism with endurance exercise
- GG variants also show significant benefit with high-intensity training including HIIT (high-intensity interval training) or moderated intervals, taking advantage of the close association between PPARG and PGC1-a
    - HIIT improves fatty acid oxidation and regulation by increasing PGC1-a and downregulating PPARG
    - HIIT increases AMPK, which activates PGC1a and then decreases PPARG

SUPPLEMENTS

- Not indicated for normal-weight individuals
- For overweight individuals – Resveratrol Extra. Take one capsule twice a day on an empty stomach.

Treating PPAR-gamma rs1801282 CG

The heterozygous coding of CG is balanced in terms of risk, and dietary treatment is the same for both normal and overweight individuals.

DIET FOR NORMAL AND OVERWEIGHT INDIVIDUALS

- Moderate caloric intake – 1,000 to 1,200 calories per day
- Lower simple carbohydrate intake (see Chapter 19 for more information)
- Maintain higher ratio of poly- or monounsaturated to saturated fat in diet
- Saturated fat to a maximum of 30 grams per day
- If you are CC for APOA2 or AA for FTO, further reduce saturated fat to 22 grams per day

EXERCISE

- CG individuals show improved glucose and insulin metabolism with endurance exercise

- CG individuals also show significant benefit with high-intensity training including HIIT or moderated intervals, taking advantage of the close association between PPARG and PGC1-a
- HIIT improves fatty acid oxidation and regulation by increasing PGC1-a and downregulating PPARG
- HIIT increases AMPK, which activates PGC1a and then decreases PPARG

SUPPLEMENTS

- For normal-weight individuals – Resveratrol Extra. Take one capsule per day on an empty stomach
- For overweight individuals – Resveratrol Extra (Pure Encapsulations). Take one capsule twice a day on an empty stomach

Treating PPAR-gamma rs1801282 CC (Risk allele)

Although C is the normal or ancestral allele, it is the one with health risks.

C is the normal allele and would have minimal risk with a more primitive, low-carbohydrate, low-calorie diet. However, the typical modern diet with high carbohydrate and fat content leads to this allele being detrimental. Therefore, maintaining a diet low in fats and simple carbohydrates is key.

C-allele

- Higher BMI
- Reduced insulin sensitivity
- Increased risk of type 2 diabetes
- Worse on a high-carbohydrate and high-saturated-fat diet
- Significant cumulative effect when combines with other polymorphisms especially FTO, TCF7L2, MC4R and APOA2
- Improved blood sugar stability with caloric reduction
- Fewer health benefits from exercise compared to GG

DIET FOR NORMAL AND OVERWEIGHT INDIVIDUALS

- Moderate caloric intake – 1,000 to 1,200 calories per day
- Limited simple carbohydrate intake (see Chapter 19 for more information)
- Maintain higher ratio of poly- or monounsaturated to saturated fat in diet
- Saturated fat to a maximum of 30 grams per day
- If you are CC for APOA2 or AA for FTO, further reduce saturated fat to 22 grams per day

EXERCISE

- Exercise still beneficial but diet is more important
- CC show moderately improved glucose and insulin metabolism with endurance exercise

SUPPLEMENTS

- For normal weight individuals – Resveratrol Extra. Take one capsule twice day on an empty stomach
- For overweight individuals – Metabolic Xtra. Take one capsule twice a day on an empty stomach

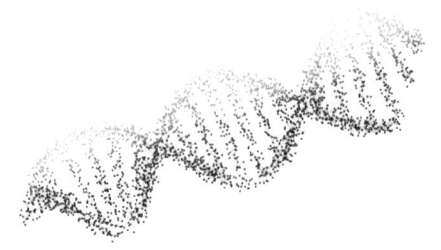

CHAPTER 12
APOA2

The Apolipoprotein Fat and Cholesterol Transport Gene
rs5082
Normal/Ancestral allele – T
Variant allele – C

APOA2 Quick Look

APOA2 C-allele – risk
- *Reduced APOA2 transcription*
- *Increased BMI when consuming a high-saturated-fat diet (>22 grams per day)*
- *Increased visceral body fat and waist circumference*
- *Increased hunger and desire for energy-dense foods resulting from increased ghrelin levels*
- *Lower efficiency of fat absorption following a meal and faster clearance from the bloodstream*
- *Lower levels of cholesterol, triglycerides, cholesterol-to-HDL ratio*
- *Lower risk of cardiovascular disease*
- *No apparent association with type 2 diabetes*

APOA2 T-allele – normal
- *No risk; ideal coding*

Note: The 23andMe platform uses plus strand terminology such that A is normal and G is variant/risk. However, the generally accepted terminology, and the one used in most research, references the minus strand such that T is normal and C is variant/risk. This is what we will use in this section. So if your 23andMe coding is A, then use T in this section. If your 23andMe coding is G, then use C.

The APOA2 gene encodes for APOlipoprotein A2, which is the second most abundant high-density lipoprotein in the body (apolipoprotein A1 is the most prevalent). Apolipoproteins A1 and A2 are the major protein components of high-density lipoproteins or HDLs, the "good cholesterol" that removes excess bad cholesterol from the blood and reduces atherosclerosis and cardiovascular disease risk. APOA2 influences the regulation of several key enzymes in lipoprotein metabolism including hepatic lipase. It also affects cholesterol ester transfer proteins, phospholipid transfer proteins, serum glucose, free fatty acid and insulin levels. It plays a significant role in modulating the body's response to dietary saturated fat.

APOA2 SNP rs5082
Normal/Ancestral allele – T
Variant/Risk allele – C

The interaction of genotype and nutrition is termed nutrigenetics. The association between the variant allele of the APOA2 gene, high BMI and a high-fat diet is one of the strongest examples of such interaction. A mean increase in BMI of 6.2% is seen in CC versus CT or TT individuals when consuming equally high amounts of saturated fat exceeding 22 grams per day. This association is of particular importance in societies with abundant food and food high in fat content (such as a typical western diet).

Compared to CT and TT, individuals with the CC genotype have been shown in multiple populations to be at a significantly increased risk of obesity when they ingest more than 22 grams of saturated fat per day. The risk is substantial with an average 6.2% increase in BMI. However, the difference does not appear to exist when fat intake is below this threshold. However, the CC genotype is also associated with increased waist circumference and visceral fat accumulation *regardless* of diet.

In addition to the metabolic effects on fat metabolism, the APOA2 C-allele also influences hunger. The C-allele predisposes to increased ghrelin levels compared to CT and TT genotypes. Ghrelin, also known as our "hunger hormone," is released by the stomach and acts on the arcuate nucleus in the hypothalamus to stimulate AGRP and NPY and stimulate the desire to seek out and consume food. This effect is most marked, as with BMI, when the individual consumes a high-fat diet. Fat, as a good fuel source, should let the stomach and then the brain know it has had enough energy to keep going for a while and should thus inhibit the release of ghrelin (our "hunger hormone"). Besides having overall higher levels of ghrelin expression, C-allele carriers also receive the opposite message. Fat intake stimulates rather than inhibits the production of ghrelin, preventing the feeling of satiety and encouraging further intake.

The C-allele is associated with slower absorption of fat from the GI tract after a meal and more rapid metabolism of fat that is absorbed. This may explain some of the other metabolic effects of the allele. Slower fat absorption and faster assimilation into storage may impair activation of satiety messengers, which, when combined with the increased levels of ghrelin, will result in prolonged feeding and increased calorific intake. It may also explain how the allele is associated with lower levels of cholesterol and triglycerides and reduced cardiovascular disease risk. Unfortunately, the downside of this improved lipid metabolism is increased intake of high-energy foods and more fat storage leading to higher visceral fat and BMI. This effect will be exacerbated by stress and cortisol, which is known to further promote visceral fat accumulation.

The association of the C-allele with a reduced risk of coronary artery disease comes from one study in an Australian population (Xiao, 2008).

TREATMENT

APOA2 The Apolipoprotein Fat and Cholesterol Transport Gene rs5082
Normal/Ancestral allele – T
Variant/Risk allele – C

Treating APOA2 rs5082 **CC**

DIET – first eight weeks

- Keep saturated fat in the diet below 22 grams per day
- Avoid high-fat keto-type diets

(For more information on fats, see sidebars on pages 103 1nd 140 and the Food Tables in Appendix 1.)

DIET – after 8 weeks

- Individuals with this coding should continue with the above recommendations after eight weeks

As with FTO, this is a very good example of why certain diets are only appropriate for certain individuals. An APOA2 C carrier following the Bulletproof Diet would have coconut oil with butter or ghee in their morning "Bulletproof coffee" and would already be over their 22 grams per day limit. They will have stimulated ghrelin, blocked leptin, slowed their metabolism and set themselves up for being hungry the rest of the day. Similar consideration would be made for versions of the Keto Diet, which recommends 80 to 125 grams of fat per day. This is why it is so important to assess your genetic metabolism before starting a new diet.

EXERCISE

- Nothing specific for this gene.

SUPPLEMENTS

- TMC. Take two capsules twice a day 30 minutes or more before lunch and dinner to regulate leptin and ghrelin. Do this for the eight-week genetic retraining period and then cycle it in one week out of every four to six weeks for maintenance.
    - If you code AA for FTO and/or CC for MC4R (other genes that have altered ghrelin and leptin activity), you may need to cycle TMC every three to four weeks rather than four to six weeks.
- Whey Satisfied Protein Powder. Put one scoop in water or almond milk at two meals a day. Note that this provides 10 grams of your protein requirement and regulates ghrelin and leptin.
- Pure Lean Fiber – a mix of soluble and insoluble fibres. Dissolve one to two scoops in water and drink it five minutes before consuming a meal likely to contain saturated fat. This supplement binds the fat to the fibre before the body absorbs it. Use this supplement *only* if you are likely to exceed the recommended 22 grams per day of saturated fat, for example, if eating out at a special function or other situations where extra fat intake is unavoidable.

Treating APOA2 rs5082 TC

DIET

- Keep saturated fat in the diet below 28 grams per day
- Avoid high-fat nutritional guides such as the Bulletproof Diet or other keto-like diets

EXERCISE

- Nothing specific for this gene

SUPPLEMENTS

- TMC. Take two capsules twice a day 30 minutes or more before lunch and dinner to regulate leptin and ghrelin. Do this for the eight-week genetic retraining period and then cycle it in one week out of every four to six weeks for maintenance.
- If you code AA for FTO and/or CC for MC4R (other genes that have altered ghrelin and leptin activity), you may need to cycle TMC every three to four weeks rather than four to six weeks.
- Whey Satisfied Protein Powder. Put one scoop in water or almond milk at two meals a day. Note that this provides 10 grams of your protein requirement and regulates ghrelin and leptin.
- Pure Lean Fiber – a mix of soluble and insoluble fibres. Dissolve one to two scoops in water and drink it five minutes before consuming a meal likely to contain saturated fat. This supplement binds the fat to the fibre before the body absorbs it. Use this supplement *only* if you are likely to exceed the recommended 22 grams per day of saturated fat, for example, if eating out at a special function or other situations where extra fat intake is unavoidable.

Treating APOA2 rs5082 TT

- Follow your genetic diet according to your other genes

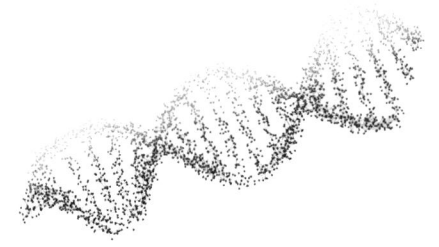

CHAPTER 13
FABP2

The Fatty Acid Binding Protein Gene
rs1799883
Normal/Ancestral allele – G
Variant allele – A

FABP2 Quick Look

FABP2 A-allele – risk
- *Increased weight gain and BMI with 53 or more grams of saturated fats per day*
- *Sensitive to high-carbohydrate intake, particularly refined sugars (such as bread and cookies)*
- *Increased glucose levels*
- *Increased insulin resistance*
- *Increased risk of type 2 diabetes*
- *Increased risk of hyperlipidemia in carriers with type 2 (but not type 1) diabetes*
- *Twice the rate of fatty acid uptake and delivery to tissue*
- *Lower HDL*
- *Higher total cholesterol*

FABP2 G-allele – normal
- *No increased risk; ideal coding*

Fatty Acid Binding Protein 2 is one of a group of proteins that play a key role in the absorption and intracellular transport of long-chain fatty acids. It is produced primarily in the small intestine and encoded by the FABP2 gene. Fatty acids are the building blocks of lipids or fats and are classified according to the number of carbon atoms in their chains or tails. Long-chain fatty acids are those with 14 or more carbon atoms. They are also classified according to the number of hydrogen bonds into saturated, monounsaturated or polyunsaturated. These fats can be found in foods as variable as dairy fat; coconut, olive, canola and safflower oils; fish oils; nuts and avocados. They include both healthy and unhealthy fats, with the nutritional value determined by a number of structural factors including length and saturation.

The ability to store fat in adipose cells was originally an evolutionary advantage, protecting the individual against starvation in times of famine. Fatty acids are key for energy production (ATP production). When compared to other macronutrients such as carbohydrates or proteins, fatty acids yield the most ATP on an energy per gram basis. This is why fatty acids are the foremost storage form of fuel in humans and animals and, to a lesser extent, in plants. Unfortunately, we are now in societies where there is often unlimited food, and this protective mechanism has backfired, leading to excess fat accumulation.

Another important factor relates to how ingested fat is metabolized. Increased fat absorption, utilization and oxidation is known to cause insulin resistance even in healthy individuals. This was possibly a protective mechanism and evolutionary advantage as it improved metabolism and prevented muscle breakdown in times of famine. However, with current dietary excesses, it is employed constantly and therefore leads to permanent metabolic changes including diabetes.

Excess fatty acids in the diet, particularly saturated ones, have a significant pro-inflammatory effect, increasing cellular mediators such as TNF-a. A high-saturated-fat meal has the potential to increase inflammation within the hypothalamus within 24 hours, causing altered sensitivity to satiety signalling molecules such as leptin and insulin. This results in hunger and is one way in which a high-calorie, fat-rich diet leads to increased dietary intake.

Adipocytes can safely store fat, but when their intracellular fat levels are excessive, the cells become inflamed and stop responding to normal hormonal signals. This is thought to be one of the key mechanisms behind the development of insulin resistance. As insulin *inhibits* lipolysis, the breakdown of fats, once adipocytes become resistant to it, lipolysis increases and they start to release more fatty acids into the bloodstream. These fatty acids are then taken up by other tissues such as the liver (leading to fatty liver) and muscle. This in turn induces insulin resistance in these tissues, further propagating the problem and accelerating the development of metabolic syndrome and its associated diseases such as type 2 diabetes, hyperlipidemia and cardiovascular disease.

FABP2 SNP rs1799883
Ala54Thr (the A-allele replaces alanine with threonine)
Normal/Ancestral allele – G
Variant/Risk allele – A

- GG – no increased sensitivity to saturated fats and sugars
- GA – approximately 25% increased sensitivity
- AA – approximately double the sensitivity

The variant A-allele codes for a fatty acid binding protein that has twice the affinity for dietary fatty acids than does the normal G-allele protein. Studies on the Arizona Pima Indian population (Baier, 2004; Formanack, 2004; Schulz 2015) found that individuals homozygous or heterozygous for the A-allele had a higher mean fasting insulin concentration, a higher insulin response to food, lower insulin-mediated glucose uptake and higher fat oxidation. Because the A-allele FABP2 protein (containing a threonine rather than alanine) has twice the affinity for long-chain fatty acids, it greatly increases their absorption and processing. This results in increased fatty acid oxidation leading to insulin resistance. The frequency of the A-allele in Pima Indians likely accounts for them having the highest reported prevalence of insulin resistance and type 2 diabetes of any population in the world. Over half the population over the age of 35 has the disease (Knowles, 1978). However, diet and exercise appear to have a profound epigenetic influence. Pima Indians with an identical genetic risk profile, living in a rural setting in the Sierra Madre Mountains of Mexico, working in fields and eating a more traditional diet than their "American-diet" influenced brethren in Arizona, have no such problem.

A study looking at native Canadians found the A-allele to be associated with significant increases in BMI and fasting plasma triglycerides (Hegele, 1996). A sibling study from Sweden revealed higher triglyceride and cholesterol levels along with increased risk of stroke (Carlsson, 2000).

A-allele carriers (homozygous AA or heterozygous GA) are far more likely to have increased serum glucose levels both after fasting and after a large meal rich in saturated fats and sugars. In addition, the amount of saturated fat consumed appears to have a profound effect on the metabolic characteristics expressed in A-allele individuals. This represents yet another example of nutrigenomics (dietary epigenetics). A study in the journal *Metabolism* (Chamberlain, 2009) found that AAs or GAs that ate a diet containing 53 grams or more of saturated fat per day had lower HDL to total cholesterol ratios; higher cholesterol, LDLs and triglycerides; and higher insulin resistance (as seen by higher levels of HOMA-IR, a biomarker of insulin resistance). The recommendation was for limited saturated fat intake in A-allele carriers.

A study from China (Xu, 2016) examining childhood obesity found a statistically higher frequency of the A-allele in the overweight/obese group when compared to normal-weight children. Blood levels of triglycerides, insulin and the HOMA-IR marker for insulin resistance were also significantly higher in these individuals. They concluded, "The FABP2 gene G54A polymorphism is related to simple children (*sic*) obesity and lipid metabolism abnormality."

An intervention study (Martinez-Lopez, 2013) looked at 109 overweight or obese adults following a **low-calorie**, low-saturated-fat diet (fat 30% with less than 7% saturated fat, protein 15%, carbohydrate 55%). After one month, those with an A-allele had significantly lower C-reactive protein, smaller waist circumference and lower waist-to-hip ratio when compared to GG genotypes. This study showed that although the variant A-allele increases risk, carriers respond more positively to dietary changes than those with the wild G-allele.

While the association of the FABP2 A-allele with fatty acid absorption and metabolism is clear, there are some population discrepancies with regard to the risk for type 2 diabetes. The majority of this arises from lack of consistency across studies including small sample sizes, ethnic differences and research methodologies. However, there is increasing evidence from multiple population studies and meta-analyses to indicate that, in most individuals, the A-allele does impart a true influence on insulin resistance and the development of type 2 diabetes.

TREATMENT
FABP2* The Fatty Acid Binding Protein Gene *rs1799882
Normal/Ancestral allele – G
Variant/Risk allele – A

Treating FABP2 **AA**

DIET – first eight weeks
- Keep saturated fat in the diet below 53 grams per day
- Avoid high-fat keto-type diets

(For more information on fats, see sidebars on pages 103 and 140 and the Food Tables in Appendix 1.)

As with FTO and APOA2, this is a very good example of why certain diets are only appropriate for certain individuals. An individual following a keto-type diet would likely exceed their daily intake of saturated fat very quickly.

There are a number of SNPs that modify FABP2 so make sure to take a look at the gene interaction summary.

DIET FOR NORMAL WEIGHT INDIVIDUALS – first eight weeks

- Lower calorie diet – 1,000 to 1,200 calories per day
- Keep simple carbohydrate intake to ½ the physical size of the protein at each meal
- Complex vegetable carbohydrates can be eaten in unlimited quantities at all meals

DIET FOR OVERWEIGHT INDIVIDUALS – first eight weeks

- Low-calorie diet – 900 to 1,100 calories per day
- Avoid simple carbohydrates at two of the three meals per day
- Simple carbohydrates can be eaten at one meal per day but limit amount to ½ the physical size of the protein for that meal
- Complex vegetable carbohydrates can be eaten in unlimited quantities at all meals

(For more information on carbohydrates, see Chapter 19 and refer to Appendix 1 Food Tables.)

DIET – after 8 weeks

- Lower calorie diet – 1,200 calories per day
- Avoid simple carbohydrates at one of the three meals per day
- Simple carbohydrates can be eaten at two meals per day but limit amount to ½ the physical size of the protein for that meal
- Complex vegetable carbohydrates can be eaten in unlimited quantities at all meals

> ### *Gene Interactions*
>
> *Look at APOA2 to further assess saturated fat intake:*
>
> - *If you code CC for APOA2, then reduce saturated fats to 22 grams per day*
> - *If you code CT for APOA2, then reduce saturated fats to 28 grams per day*
>
> *You also need to look at TCF7L2 and IRS1 for carbohydrate intake:*
>
> - *If you are homozygote variant for TCF7L2 (TT) and/or homozygote variant for IRS1 (CC), then you need to reduce carbohydrate consumption further. Limit intake of simple carbohydrates to ½ the physical size of the protein at only one meal per day instead of three meals. This applies to both normal and overweight individuals on an ongoing basis.*
> - *If you are heterozygote for TCF7L2 (CT) and/or heterozygote for IRS1 (TC), then you need to reduce carbohydrate consumption slightly. Limit intake of simple carbohydrates to ½ the physical size of the protein at two meals per day instead of three meals. This applies to both normal and overweight individuals on an ongoing basis.*
> - *Complex vegetable carbohydrates can be eaten in unlimited quantities at all meals.*

EXERCISE

- No specific recommendations.

SUPPLEMENTS

- Whey Satisfied Protein Powder. Put one scoop in water or almond milk and drink at two meals a day. Note that this

provides 10 grams of your protein requirement and regulates ghrelin and leptin.
- If you are prone to unstable blood sugar (get light-headed or dizzy, anxious or "hangry," or feel hungry quickly)
  - Metabolic Xtra. Take one capsule twice a day on an empty stomach.
- Pure Lean Fiber – a mix of soluble and insoluble fibres. Dissolve one to two scoops in water and drink five minutes before consuming a meal likely to contain saturated fat. This supplement binds the fat to the fibre before the body absorbs it. Use this supplement *only* if you are likely to exceed your recommended saturated fat allowance, for example, if eating out at a special function or other situations where extra fat intake is unavoidable.

Treating FABP2 **GA**

DIET – first eight weeks

- Keep saturated fat in the diet below 53 grams per day
- Avoid high-fat keto-type diets

DIET FOR NORMAL-WEIGHT INDIVIDUALS – first eight weeks

- Lower calorie diet – 1,200 to 1,300 calories per day
- Keep simple carbohydrate intake to ½ the physical size of the protein at each meal
- Complex vegetable carbohydrates can be eaten in unlimited quantities at all meals

DIET FOR OVERWEIGHT INDIVIDUALS – first eight weeks

- Low-calorie diet – 1,000 to 1,200 calories per day
- Avoid simple carbohydrates at two of the three meals per day

- Simple carbohydrates can be eaten at one meal per day but limit amount to ½ the physical size of the protein for that meal
- Complex vegetable carbohydrates can be eaten in unlimited quantities at all meals

(For more information on carbohydrates, see Chapter 19 and refer to Appendix 1 Food Tables.)

DIET – after 8 weeks

- Lower calorie diet – 1,200 to 1,300 calories per day
- Avoid simple carbohydrates at one of the three meals per day
- Simple carbohydrates can be eaten at two meals per day but limit amount to ½ the physical size of the protein for that meal
- Complex vegetable carbohydrates can be eaten in unlimited quantities at all meals

EXERCISE

- No specific recommendations

SUPPLEMENTS

- Whey Satisfied Protein Powder. Put one scoop in water or almond milk and drink at two meals a day. Note that this provides 10 grams of your protein requirement and regulates ghrelin and leptin.
- If you are prone to unstable blood sugar (get light-headed or dizzy, anxious or "hangry," or feel hungry quickly):
  - Metabolic Xtra. Take one capsule twice a day on an empty stomach.
- Pure Lean Fiber – a mix of soluble and insoluble fibers. Dissolve one to two scoops dissolved in water and drink five minutes before consuming a meal likely to contain saturated fat. This supplement binds the fat to the fibre before the body absorbs it. Use this supplement *only* if you are likely to exceed your recommended saturated fat allowance, for example, if eating

out at a special function or other situations where extra fat intake is unavoidable.

> **Gene Interactions**
>
> Look at APOA2 to further assess saturated fat intake:
>
> - If you code CC for APOA2, then reduce saturated fats to 22 grams per day
> - If you code CT for APOA2, then reduce saturated fats to 28 grams per day
>
> You also need to look at TCF7L2 and IRS1 for carbohydrate intake:
>
> - If you are homozygote variant for TCF7L2 (TT) and/or homozygote variant for IRS1 (CC), then you need to reduce carbohydrate consumption further. Limit intake of simple carbohydrates to ½ the physical size of the protein at only one meal per day instead of three meals. This applies to both normal and overweight individuals on an ongoing basis.
> - If you are heterozygote for TCF7L2 (CT) and/or heterozygote for IRS1 (TC), then you need to reduce carbohydrate consumption slightly. Limit intake of simple carbohydrates to ½ the physical size of the protein at two meals per day instead of three meals. This applies to both normal and overweight individuals on an ongoing basis.
> - Complex vegetable carbohydrates can be eaten in unlimited quantities at all meals.

Treating FABP2 **GG**

DIET

- Follow your genetic diet according to your other genes

EXERCISE

- No specific recommendations

SUPPLEMENTS

- None recommended

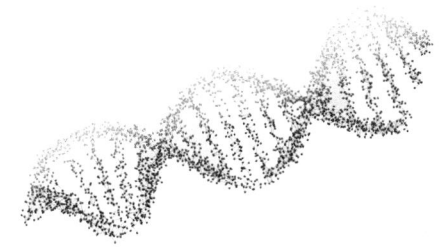

CHAPTER 14
TCF7L2

The Blood Sugar Stabilizing Gene
rs17903146
Normal/Ancestral allele – C
Variant allele – T

TCF7L2 Quick Look

TCF7L2 T-allele – risk
- *Increased risk of type 2 diabetes: twofold for TT and 1.4-fold for CT*
- *Increased weight gain and higher BMI*
- *Increased sensitivity to carbohydrate and saturated fat intake*
- *Altered glucose and insulin levels*
- *Increased risk for metabolic syndrome*
- *Increased abdominal adiposity*
- *Increased colon cancer risk*
- *Increased risk of cardiovascular disease*

TCF7L2 C-allele – normal
- *No increased risk; ideal coding*

TCF7L2 or TransCription Factor 7-Like 2 codes for the protein T-cell transcription factor 4 (TCF4) and is highly implicated in blood glucose homeostasis. It alters the expression of other genes that control insulin after the consumption of carbohydrates and saturated fats. It may act through the control of pro-glucagon (the complementary hormone to insulin) via the Wnt signalling pathway. (Wnt is an acronym in the genetic world for Wingless/Integrated.) This is a group of evolutionarily ancient signal transduction pathways that pass signals into cells via surface receptors. It is strongly associated with pancreatic beta-cell dysfunction.

The SNP rs7903146 is one of two SNPs linked with TCF7L2, the other being rs4506565. They are both strongly implicated in the development of type 2 diabetes with a correlation of 92%. SNPR rs7903146 is the stronger of the two in terms of etiological association.

TCF7L2 SNP rs17903146
Normal/Ancestral allele – C
Variant/Risk allele – T

The T-allele is strongly linked to the development of type 2 diabetes across multiple populations. Numerous studies have demonstrated that the SNP increases population-attributable risk by 16 to 21%. Heterozygous (TC) individuals have a Relative Risk of 1.45 while the homozygous genotype (CC) confers a Relative Risk of 2.41.

The T-allele is also implicated in gestational diabetes and increased birth weight. This effect is likely mediated by reduced maternal insulin secretion during pregnancy and therefore higher blood glucose levels. A study published in *The American Journal of Human Genetics* (Freathy, 2007) found an 18-gram increase in birth weight per maternal T-allele.

The T-allele is very strong predictor for the future development of type 2 diabetes. The variant allele leads to overexpression of TCF7L2 in pancreatic islets (beta-cells), which reduces glucose-stimulated insulin release. Carriers of the allele have impaired insulin secretion and impaired response to dietary glucose intake. They also demonstrate significantly higher glucose production by the liver.

A study from 2012 (Phillips, 2012) found that female T-allele carriers had increased risk of metabolic syndrome (Odds Ratio 1.66), elevated insulin levels and insulin resistance, increased BMI and adiposity, and higher blood pressure compared to CC homozygotes. The study also found there to be a strong epigenetic dietary component. High-saturated fat intake increased the Odds Ratio of metabolic syndrome from 1.66 to 2.35 and was associated with further impairment of insulin sensitivity.

Another study (Corella, 2013) found that adherence to a Mediterranean diet (high unsaturated fats and complex carbohydrates) resulted in markedly reduced fasting glucose and lipids and a lower incidence of stroke. Ouhaibi-Djellouli (2014) found that high-dessert intake was correlated with increased expression of the TT genotype while Hindy (2012) found high-fibre intake to reduce its influence.

As with adults, the T-allele has been shown to impair glucose metabolism and possibly increase risk of type 2 diabetes in obese children.

The T-allele for TCF7L2 is associated with increased rates of colon cancer. A prospective cohort study of over 13,000 U.S. adults (Folsom, 2008) found that individuals homozygous for the T-allele were twice as likely to develop colon cancer as those with a CC genotype. Among white subjects, there was also a 50% increase in risk of lung cancer. These findings appear to be an independent effect of the T-allele not explained by the increased risk of type 2 diabetes. The link between TCF7L2 and colon cancer is not fully understood but, as with diabetic risk, may be linked to alterations in the Wnt system. The gene plays a central role in the Wnt/β-catenin signalling pathway, which is strongly implicated in colon cancer etiology. Mutations in the adenomatous polyposis coli (*APC*) gene cause colon cancer via this pathway. Mutations in either *APC* or genes that modulate β-catenin can alter this regulatory relationship and lead to the activation or inhibition of genes that contribute to neoplasia.

There is a significant association between the T-allele and cardiovascular disease. One study (Sousa, 2009) found that the variant allele in both diabetic and non-diabetic subjects increased risk and severity of coronary artery disease and cardiovascular events including stroke and heart attack.

TREATMENT

TCF7L2 The Blood Sugar Stabilizing Gene rs7903146
Normal/Ancestral allele – C
Variant/Risk allele – T

Treating TCF7L2 TT

DIET – first eight weeks

For all TT carriers, regardless of weight:

- Avoid simple carbohydrates at two of the three meals per day
- Simple carbohydrates can be eaten at one meal per day but limit the amount to ½ the physical size of the protein for that meal. Simple carbohydrates include grains (breads, pastas, rice, corn, popcorn, legumes, quinoa, etc.), starches (potato, sweet potato, yam, squash, etc.), sweets, fruits or alcohol.
    - If you code variant CC for IRS1 and/or variant AA for FTO, then it becomes even more important that you adhere to the above guidelines for TCF7L2
- Complex vegetable and salad carbohydrates can be eaten in unlimited quantities at all meals
- Lower saturated fats in the diet to less than 30 to 35 grams per day
    - If you are homozygote variant CC for APOA2, then your saturated fat content needs to be reduced to 22 grams per day

- If you are heterozygote TC for APOA2, then your saturated fat content needs to be reduced to 28 grams per day

Diet – after 8 weeks

- Avoid simple carbohydrates at one of the three meals per day
- Simple carbohydrates can be eaten at two meals per day but limit the amount to ½ the physical size of the protein for that meal. Simple carbohydrates include grains (breads, pastas, rice, corn, popcorn, legumes, quinoa, etc.), starches (potato, sweet potato, yam, squash, etc.), sweets, fruits or alcohol.
- Complex vegetable carbohydrates can be eaten in unlimited quantities at all meals
- Lower saturated fats in the diet to less than 30 to 35 grams per day
    - If you are homozygote variant CC for APOA2, then your saturated fat content needs to be reduced to 22 grams per day
    - If you are heterozygote TC for APOA2, then your saturated fat content needs to be reduced to 28 grams per day

---

Gene Interactions

Look at IRS1 and FTO to further assess carbohydrate intake:

- *If you code variant CC for IRS1 and/or variant AA for FTO, then it becomes even more important that you adhere to the above guidelines for TCF7L2*

Look at APOA2 to further assess your saturated fat intake:

- *If you are homozygote variant CC for APOA2, then your saturated fat content needs to be reduced to 22 grams per day*
- *If you are heterozygote TC for APOA2, then your saturated fat content needs to be reduced to 28 grams per day*

EXERCISE

- Diet appears to be the most important epigenetic factor with TCF7L2
- Regular exercise is to be encouraged for its ability to improve handling of blood sugar, reduced insulin requirement and lower cardiovascular disease risk

SUPPLEMENTS

- If you are prone to unstable blood sugar (get light-headed or dizzy, anxious or "hangry," or feel hungry quickly):
  - Metabolic Xtra. Take one capsule twice a day on an empty stomach
- Pure Lean Fiber — a mix of soluble and insoluble fibres. Dissolve one to two scoops in water and drink five minutes before consuming a meal likely to contain saturated fat. This supplement binds the fat to the fibre before the body absorbs it. Use this supplement *only* if you are likely to exceed your recommended saturated fat allowance, for example, if eating out at a special function or other situations where extra fat intake is unavoidable.

Treating TCF7L2 rs7903146 CT

DIET – first eight weeks

For all CT carriers, regardless of weight:

- Avoid simple carbohydrates at one of the three meals per day
- Simple carbohydrates can be eaten at two meals per day but limit the amount to ½ the physical size of the protein for that meal. Simple carbohydrates include grains (breads, pastas, rice, corn, popcorn, legumes, quinoa, etc.), starches (potato, sweet potato, yam, squash, etc.), sweets, fruits or alcohol.

- If you code variant CC for IRS1 and/or variant AA for FTO, then it becomes even more important that you adhere to the above guidelines for TCF7L2
- Complex vegetable and salad carbohydrates can be eaten in unlimited quantities at all meals
- Lower saturated fats in the diet to less than 30 to 35 grams per day
  - If you are homozygote variant CC for APOA2, then your saturated fat content needs to be reduced to 22 grams per day
  - If you are heterozygote TC for APOA2, then your saturated fat content needs to be reduced to 28 grams per day

Diet – after 8 weeks

- Simple carbohydrates can be eaten at all meals per day but limit the amount to ½ the physical size of the protein for that meal. Simple carbohydrates include grains (breads, pastas, rice, corn, popcorn, legumes, quinoa, etc.), starches (potato, sweet potato, yam, squash, etc.), sweets, fruits or alcohol.
- Complex vegetable carbohydrates can be eaten in unlimited quantities at all meals
- Lower saturated fats in the diet to less than 30 to 35 grams per day

EXERCISE

- Diet appears to be the most important epigenetic factor with TCF7L2
- Regular exercise is to be encouraged for its ability to improve handling of blood sugar, reduce insulin requirement and lower cardiovascular disease risk

SUPPLEMENTS

- If you are prone to unstable blood sugar (get light-headed or dizzy, anxious or "hangry," or feel hungry quickly):

- ○ Metabolic Xtra. Take one capsule twice a day on an empty stomach
- Pure Lean Fiber – a mix of soluble and insoluble fibres. Dissolve one to two scoops in water and drink five minutes before consuming a meal likely to contain saturated fat. This supplement binds the fat to the fibre before the body absorbs it. Use this supplement *only* if you are likely to exceed your recommended saturated fat allowance, for example, if eating out at a special function or other situations where extra fat intake is unavoidable.

Treating TCF7L2 rs7903146 CC

DIET

- Eat a diet according to your other genes

EXERCISE

- Regular exercise is to be encouraged for its ability to improve handling of blood sugar, reduce insulin requirement and lower cardiovascular disease risk

SUPPLEMENTS

- None recommended

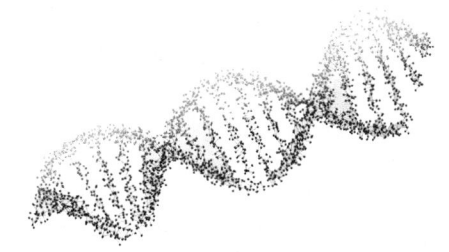

CHAPTER 15
IRS1

The Insulin Receptor Gene
rs2943641
Normal/Ancestral allele – T
Variant allele – C

IRS1 Quick Look

IRS1 C-allele – risk

- *Increased insulin resistance*
- *Increased glucose levels*
- *Lower body fat but increased proportion of visceral fat in men*
- *Decreased adiponectin*
- *Reduced HDL and increased TGs*
- *Increased type 2 diabetes*
- *Increased risk of metabolic syndrome*

IRS1 T-allele – normal
- *No increased risk; ideal coding*
- *Lowered risk of insulin resistance, type 2 diabetes and metabolic syndrome*

The gene IRS1 codes for the protein Insulin Receptor Substrate 1, which plays a key role in the insulin receptor signal transduction pathway and the cellular effects of insulin. IRS1 is one of the major proteins initiating an intracellular cascade that increases glucose transport in both muscle and adipose tissue. IRS1 is considered a docking protein that binds to insulin and IGF-1 receptors and undergoes tyrosine phosphorylation resulting in activation of a multitude of signalling pathways and increased glucose uptake. Blocking of the IRS1 induced pathway by inflammatory mediators such as TNF-α may be one mechanism by which inflammation leads to insulin resistance. Persistently high blood sugar also causes biochemical modification of the IRS1 protein, impairing its function and further increasing insulin resistance. IRS1 deficiency-related insulin resistance also leads to hypertension and hyperlipidemia.

IRS1 plays a key role in transmitting signals from insulin and insulin-like growth factor-1 (IGF-1) receptors to pathways inside of the cells. The phosphorylation associated with this protein is absent in tissues lacking IRS1. Numerous polymorphisms in this gene are associated with type II diabetes and susceptibility to insulin resistance with rs2942641 being one of the most established in terms of research.

Along with other SNPs at the same IRS1 gene locus, the rs2943641 variant (C) allele is associated with an increased ratio of visceral to subcutaneous fat, insulin resistance, metabolic syndrome, poor lipid profile, and increased risk of type 2 diabetes and coronary artery disease.

The IRS1 gene interacts with PI3K pathways. PI3K, or phosphatidylinositol 3-kinase, is part of a family of enzymes involved in cellular functions such as cellular growth, proliferation, differentiation and motility, all of which are turned on in cancer. Mice bred without the IRS1 gene show significant growth retardation. A number of nuclear functions have been linked to IRS1 including DNA repair, transcription activity and cellular growth, all of which are important in carcinogenesis. Its precise role, however, is unclear, with both over- and under-expression being linked to different types of cancer. In the majority of cases, increased expression is associated with poor outcome including acute lymphoblastic leukemia; and breast, hepatic, prostate and colorectal cancer. Under-expression is thought to increase risk of non-small cell lung cancer. This specific IRS1/P13K interaction is involved in the insulin and glucose insensitivity of cancerous tumours and their response to calorie restriction.

IRS1 SNP rs2943641
Normal/Ancestral allele – T
Variant/Risk allele – C

For this SNP, the normal or ancestral allele, T, is actually the **minor** allele, meaning it is less common in most populations than the variant or risk allele, C.

(This IRS1 SNP should not be confused with other IRS1 SNPs such as rs1801278 [Gly972Arg] and rs1801276 [Ala513Pro], which are also implicated in insulin resistance and glucose metabolism but have more variable research support.)

The risk allele C is associated with:

- Decreased IRS1 protein production and phosphorylation
- Increased insulin resistance
- Increased glucose levels
- Lower body fat but increased proportion of visceral fat in men
- Decreased adiponectin
- Reduced HDL and increased TGs
- Increased type 2 diabetes
- Increased metabolic syndrome
- Possible hypertension
- Increased inflammation
- Possible increased cancer risk in obese individuals

The variant C-allele is significantly associated with an increased risk of type 2 diabetes in multiple populations. Rung (2009) found the

C-allele to increase type 2 diabetes risk by 19% in a Scandinavian population. Yiannakouris (2012) found the CC variant to increase risk by 6% in European individuals, and Ohshige (2011), looking at Japanese subjects, found an increased risk of 21%. Zheng (2013) calculated a type 2 diabetes Odds Ratio of 1.69 for C-allele carriers with increased risk of insulin resistance and metabolic syndrome in two independent populations. The Odds Ratio for type 2 diabetes in the Saudi population was found to be 1.48 (Alharbi, 2014).

Interestingly, a study looking at subjects in Bosnia and Herzegovina (Mahmutovic, 2019), a population with a high prevalence of type 2 diabetes, found the C-allele to be associated with lower fasting blood sugar and HbA1c (a measure of glucose control), indicating the importance of other genes and dietary factors particularly in this demographic.

While reducing overall adiposity, the C-allele increases the ratio of visceral to subcutaneous fat, a risk factor for insulin resistance, type 2 diabetes and metabolic syndrome. It also confers a less favourable lipid profile, reducing HDL and increasing triglycerides (Kilpelainen, 2011).

The normal T-allele confers a 6% lower risk of type 2 diabetes and an Odds Ratio of 0.89 compared to CC. In addition, genome-wide association studies also showed that the T-allele is associated with lower fasting insulin and better post-glucose insulin homeostasis. Overall the T-allele is associated with improved handling and response to carbohydrate load.

Of particular importance for this gene SNP is the influence of dietary fat and carbohydrate. An interventional weight-loss study by Qi (Qi, 2011) looking at how diet can influence the metabolic effect of SNP genotypes concluded that CC individuals responded best to a diet with a lower saturated fat-to-carbohydrate ratio. At first glance, it appears that the CC individuals lost more weight, had lower insulin and less insulin resistance when assigned to a *high-carbohydrate* diet, which is somewhat paradoxical given what is known about the gene and its association with diabetes. However, closer inspection and interpretation of their discussion reveals that all participants were essentially on a low *simple* carbohydrate diet. That is, their carbohydrate intake was restricted to complex, low-glycemic options. As such, changes in percentage of energy intake were more a reflection of lower fat intake than increased carbohydrates. The combination of low saturated fat and low high-glycemic carbs resulted in the best overall outcome for CC individuals. It should also be noted that this was a weight-loss study looking at a population already showing the effects of high BMI.

In a similar study, and of equal importance, Zheng (2013) found that the beneficial effects of the T-allele were maximized when individuals restricted saturated fat intake. He also found that a more western diet containing higher glycemic carbohydrates was detrimental to C-allele carriers. Another study by Ericson (2013) indicated a significant difference between sexes, with female T-allele carriers doing better with lower carb and higher fat intake, while men had more effect with higher carb and lower fat.

Much of the inconsistency in these studies arises as a result of significant differences in study populations and dietary regimens including choice and ratios of carbohydrates and fats. My recommendations are based on a combination of research and experience with my own patient population. In addition, this is one of the many examples where gene interaction plays a considerable role, and the effects of other SNPs need to be integrated into management.

A number of nuclear functions have been linked to IRS1 including DNA repair, transcription activity and cellular growth, all of which are important in carcinogenesis. In addition, obesity and insulin resistance are associated with increased risk of some cancers. IRS1, as a signalling adapter protein able to integrate different signalling cascades from other pathways, may play a role in cancer progression with high-carbohydrate consumption. Obese individuals with the T-allele demonstrated significantly lower risk of cancer in one Swedish study (Maglio, 2013). Although IRS1 expression has been correlated with numerous cancer types, the role of specific SNPs in overall risk has not been clearly established. There appears to be some increased risk of colorectal, breast and prostate cancer associated with the rs1801278 SNP, but this has not been established for rs2943641.

TREATMENT

IRS1 The Insulin Receptor Gene rs2943641
Normal/Ancestral allele – T
Variant/Risk allele – C

For this SNP, the normal or ancestral allele, T, is actually the minor allele, meaning it is less common in most populations than is the variant or risk allele, C.

Treating IRS1 **CC**

DIET – first eight weeks

For all CC carriers, regardless of weight:

- Avoid simple carbohydrates at two of the three meals per day
- Simple carbohydrates can be eaten at one meal per day but limit the amount to ½ the physical size of the protein for that meal. Simple carbohydrates include grains (breads, pastas, rice, corn, popcorn, legumes, quinoa, etc.), starches (potato, sweet potato, yam, squash, etc.), sweets, fruits or alcohol.
    - If you code variant CC for TCF7L2 TT and/or variant AA for FTO, then it becomes even more important that you adhere to the above guidelines for IRS1
- Complex vegetable and salad carbohydrates can be eaten in unlimited quantities at all meals
- Lower saturated fats in the diet to less than 28 grams per day

- If you are homozygote variant CC for APOA2, then your saturated fat content needs to be reduced to 22 grams per day

Diet – after 8 weeks

- Avoid simple carbohydrates at one of the three meals per day
- Simple carbohydrates can be eaten at two meals per day but limit the amount to ½ the physical size of the protein for that meal. Simple carbohydrates include grains (breads, pastas, rice, corn, popcorn, legumes, quinoa, etc.), starches (potato, sweet potato, yam, squash, etc.), sweets, fruits or alcohol.
- Complex vegetable carbohydrates can be eaten in unlimited quantities at all meals
- Lower saturated fats in the diet to less than 28 grams per day
  - If you are homozygote variant CC for APOA2, then your saturated fat content needs to be reduced to 22 grams per day

---

Gene Interactions

Look at TCF7L2 and FTO to further assess carbohydrate intake:

- *If you code variant TT for TCF7L2 and/or variant AA for FTO, then it becomes even more important that you adhere to the above guidelines for IRS1*

Look at APOA2 to further assess fat intake:

- *If you code variant CC for APOA2, then keep saturated fats below 22 grams per day*

EXERCISE

- Diet appears to be the most important epigenetic factor with IRS1
- Regular exercise is to be encouraged for its ability to improve handling of blood sugar, reduce insulin requirement and lower cardiovascular disease risk

SUPPLEMENTS

- If you are prone to unstable blood sugar (get light-headed or dizzy, anxious or "hangry," or feel hungry quickly):
  - Metabolic Xtra. Take one capsule twice a day on an empty stomach
- Vitamin D. Take 1,000 IU per day, as research indicates improved insulin sensitivity and reduced type 2 diabetes risk

Treating IRS1 rs2943641 TC

DIET – first eight weeks

For all TC carriers, regardless of weight:

- Avoid simple carbohydrates at one of the three meals per day
- Simple carbohydrates can be eaten at two meals per day but limit the amount to ½ the physical size of the protein for that meal. Simple carbohydrates include grains (breads, pastas, rice, corn, popcorn, legumes, quinoa, etc.), starches (potato, sweet potato, yam, squash, etc.), sweets, fruits or alcohol.
  - If you code variant CC for TCF7L2 TT and/or variant AA for FTO, then it becomes even more important that you adhere to the above guidelines for IRS1
- Complex vegetable and salad carbohydrates can be eaten in unlimited quantities at all meals
- Lower saturated fats in the diet to less than 28 grams per day

- - If you are homozygote variant CC for APOA2, then your saturated fat content needs to be reduced to 22 grams per day

Diet – after 8 weeks

- Simple carbohydrates can be eaten at all meals per day but limit the amount to ½ the physical size of the protein for that meal. Simple carbohydrates include grains (breads, pastas, rice, corn, popcorn, legumes, quinoa, etc.), starches (potato, sweet potato, yam, squash, etc.), sweets, fruits or alcohol.
- Complex vegetable carbohydrates can be eaten in unlimited quantities at all meals
- Lower saturated fats in the diet to less than 28 grams per day
  - If you are homozygote variant CC for APOA2, then your saturated fat content needs to be reduced to 22 grams per day

EXERCISE

- Diet appears to be the most important epigenetic factor with IRS1
- Regular exercise is to be encouraged for its ability to improve handling of blood sugar, reduce insulin requirement and lower cardiovascular disease risk

SUPPLEMENTS

- If you are prone to unstable blood sugar (get light headed or dizzy, anxious or "hangry," or feel hungry quickly):
  - Metabolic Xtra. Take one capsule twice a day on an empty stomach
- Vitamin D. Take 1,000 IU per day, as research indicates improved insulin sensitivity and reduced type 2 diabetes risk

Treating IRS1 rs29427641 **TT**

- Although this coding means you have a lower risk of insulin resistance, type 2 diabetes and metabolic syndrome, there is evidence that this effect is reduced if your diet has a high total fat or saturated fat-to-carbohydrate ratio. Therefore, I recommend keeping your saturated fat below 30 to 35 grams per day and avoid fat-dense diets such as keto diets
- Although carbohydrates are not limited, I recommend sticking to low-glycemic complex sources to maximize the benefit of your coding
- Women with TT can increase their fat intake a little (about 35 to 40 grams per day) *unless* contraindicated by APOA2
  - If you are homozygote variant CC for APOA2, then your saturated fat content needs to be reduced to 22 grams per day
  - If you are heterozygote TC for APOA2, then your saturated fat content needs to be reduced to 28 grams per day
- Men can increase their carbohydrate intake a little unless variant (TT) for TCF7L2

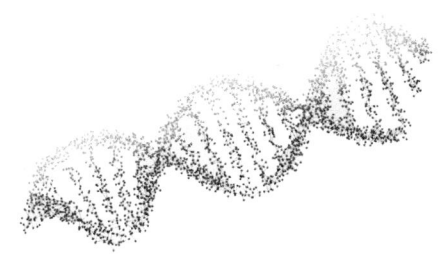

CHAPTER 16
Case Study #4
Carbohydrates and Inflammation

Larry is an 82-year-old retired teacher with osteoarthritis affecting his hands, knees and low back. He had been a long-term user of anti-inflammatory medication, but he had weaned himself off on the advice of his family doctor in order to avoid possible side effects. Over the past few years, he had managed to control the inflammation, pain and stiffness through simple changes to his diet and lifestyle. This included strengthening and mobility exercises, weight loss and avoidance of "deadly nightshade" foods such as potatoes, eggplant, tomato and peppers.

Sadly, his wife became sick, and he noticed that the stress this caused brought back all his old symptoms: stiff, achy joints in the morning; pain and swelling throughout the day; and a marked deterioration in his abilities to carry out daily chores and provide care. He realized the role stress was playing in his symptoms and tried meditation, counselling and relaxation therapy. Although he was feeling and sleeping better, his joints were still bothersome, and he felt fatigued during the day.

He had already pulled out all deadly nightshades, red meat and dairy products before seeing me, which had only made a small dent in his pain.

During my consultation with Larry, we discussed his diet. He had continued to avoid the deadly nightshade foods and, in addition, had cut back on red meat and dairy. However, he reported that with his wife being unwell, he had to prepare most meals and had defaulted to more pastas and grains for convenience. His fresh vegetables were limited and he had replaced these with fruit.

Larry's genetic profile included the following coding:

- TCF7L2 – CT: increased insulin resistance and weight gain with moderate- to high-carbohydrate intake
- IRS1 – CC: increased insulin resistance, diabetes risk and inflammation
- ADRB2 – GG: increased stress response and inflammatory response
- FTO: moderate carbohydrate sensitivity, requiring average protein intake
- MCM6* – AA: no adverse reaction to dairy products

This SNP is not included in the book but is a part of my workup in this case.

Larry's genetic coding meant that he responded poorly to the increased carbohydrate in his diet. Besides increasing his risk of diabetes and weight gain (not ideal for his joints), carbohydrates increased his overall level of inflammation. This was further aggravated by his exaggerated inflammatory response to stress. Interestingly, in this case, one of Larry's other gene codings indicated that he actually handled dairy products quite well and did not need to exclude them from his diet.

Based on his genetics, I recommended he reduce his carbohydrate intake by eliminating all high-glycemic carbohydrates such as sugars, white refined foods and fruits except berries. Vegetables and salads were allowed in unlimited quantities at all meals. High-carbohydrate, low-glycemic foods such as wild rice, sweet potato, legumes and berries were only allowed at two of his three meals per day. The amount of carbohydrate at these meals was only to be ½ the physical size of the protein portion.

I allowed him to reintroduce dairy products in the form of high-protein, plain, non-sweetened Greek yogurt and cottage cheese as added protein sources. I encouraged him to eat more fish in his diet rather than red meat and to add in other anti-inflammatory omega-3 fat sources such as walnuts, olives and avocados.

I recommended the following supplements (see Appendix 2) to help reduce inflammation and repair his joints:
- Arthoben – 1½ tablespoons in water twice a day
- Resveratrol Extra – one capsule twice a day
- Liposomal Glutathione and NAC – one capsule of each twice a day

Three weeks later Larry found the mobility in his hands improving, and the pain in his knees had decreased by approximately 40%. By six weeks, he reported improvement in pain, swelling and stiffness of about 90%, allowing significantly more activity in his daily life. His overall energy levels were better, with less fatigue and weakness. At the eight-week mark, I reduced his Resveratrol, Liposomal Glutathione and NAC to one capsule of each per day but the Arthoben to 1½ tablespoons once a day.

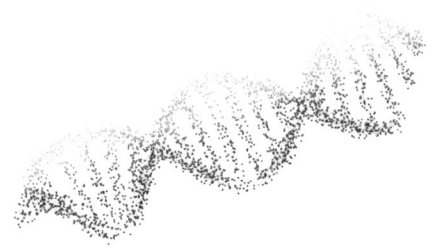

CHAPTER 17

The Stress Genes

ADRB2, NR3C2, CRHR1 and FKBP5
The Impact of Stress on Gene Expression and How This Is Affected by SNP Coding

Everyone is familiar with the scenario typically used to teach the principles of stress. Prehistoric man is meandering along and minding his own business, wondering whether to wear the bison or the bearskin loincloth for dinner, when a sabre-tooth tiger leaps out of the bushes. The "fight-or-flight" mechanism is activated. Adrenaline kicks in, causing pupils to dilate, heart and breathing rate to jump, the skin to go cold and the hair to stand up. Muscles twitch in anticipation of the next move, and senses are heightened. The man throws a rock, then jumps quickly into a gully, running as fast as he can, powered by the surge of increased energy and blood sugar. By now, cortisol, the major stress hormone, is beginning to rise, supporting the initial adrenalin rush to permit a prolonged reaction to the inherent danger. It is more potent and long-lasting with profound effects at the cellular level. In moments the threat is over. The tiger has found more accessible prey. He sighs in relief, the danger past and his cave in sight, and the man's alarm system turns off. The stress hormones stabilize his body before switching off and returning to normal levels. The mechanism has worked. It has enabled survival through danger and restored life to normal with no ill effects apart from a battered prehistoric ego!

What is less familiar is the scenario 3,000 years later.

"Downtown man," tired from a sleepless night, has already battled with what he perceives as the first "stressful situation" of the day—whether to wear the Armani or Prada power suit to the merger presentation—and is now sitting in traffic, 15 minutes late for work. His mobile phone rings. It's his boss, informing him that if he's late, he might as well not show up at all. Reaching to put the phone down, he knocks his coffee over onto the presentation sheets on the passenger seat. The traffic hasn't moved an inch. Despite the fact that none of this is anywhere near as dangerous as a sabre-toothed tiger, his brain is programmed to interpret such situations as "stressful." Unfortunately, the primitive areas of the brain and associated hormone reactions have not progressed much since his loincloth days. The "fight-or-flight" mechanism kicks into action. The cascade of adrenalin and cortisol begins, raising heart rate, blood pressure and breathing. Unfortunately, unlike the first scenario, "downtown man's" stressful situation does not resolve quickly and when it does, another rapidly replaces it. The stress reaction continually battles to restore a "safe" normality that does not exist.

Chronic stimulation of the stress reaction leads to hormonal and metabolic imbalances that adversely affect all systems in the body. These range from the well-recognized effects on metabolism and weight termed *Metabolic Syndrome* and the reduction in athletic performance seen in *Overtraining Syndrome* to impairment of fertility, immunity and healing. The main culprit is cortisol, the stress hormone that supports a prolonged and powerful "fight-or-flight" reaction. Its action, of necessity for its primary role, reaches all tissues of the body. Unfortunately, in excess, its harmful effects are equally as far reaching.

The pervasiveness of chronic stress in our 21st century society is no longer a surprise to most people. What may have been the subject of an occasional editorial is now emblazoned over every magazine cover and is likely the most frequent topic of talk shows and health programs. We have become somewhat immune to statistics such as 80 to 90% of visits to doctors' offices are due to stress or stress-related disorders, or 45% of teens and 26% of tweens report being anxious.

We skip over reports that tranquilizers, anti-depressants and anti-anxiety medications account for 25% of all prescriptions written. All of this is true, and it probably represents the most serious health crisis of our generation. However, the pervasiveness of stress means we ignore it. Unfortunately, that may have a lasting effect on generations to come, not simply because the burden of treating many stress-related diseases will fall upon our younger population, but because it appears our chronic stress is changing our genes in a way that is detrimental to our children even if they do manage to remain stress-free.

The rapidly expanding field of epigenetics examines how modification of genetic expression rather than genetic code can influence health and disease. Lifestyle factors such as diet and exercise can modify transcription of certain genes by enzymatically attaching a chemical tag (most commonly a methyl group). Epigenetic tags can be added or deleted through generations. One factor that exerts a profound influence on gene expression is chronic stress, with new research indicating that alterations in function may be inheritable.

In a study from Emory University School of Medicine in Atlanta (Dias, 2014), rats conditioned to respond fearfully to the smell of acetophenone passed this trait on to subsequent generations. The grandchildren expressed more smell receptors and had a similar epigenetic marker to their grandparents.

Similarly in humans, researchers in New York analyzed the genes of Jewish subjects interned in concentration camps who witnessed or experienced torture, or who were forced to hide during the Second World War, as well as the genes of their children. The children had significantly higher levels of anxiety and stress disorders. Epigenetic tags were found on genes associated with trauma and stress in the Holocaust survivors and their offspring but were not in a control group (Yehuda, 2016).

These are two examples of epigenetic inheritance, whereby altered gene expression is inherited in the same way as genetic code. It has profound implications in terms of health. Factors such as stress, poor diet and exposure to toxins that have a detrimental effect on one generation can be passed on to the next. The accumulation of genetic dysfunction over multiple generations will inevitably lead to progressively deteriorating health and increased incidence of disease.

Cortisol, our stress hormone, is able to cross the nuclear membrane of cells, bind to mRNA, change transcription and alter DNA replication. It can create new SNPs as well as activate or suppress existing ones. Researchers looking at the effect of stress and cortisol on genes related to the immune system found this epigenetic factor alters the expression of over 2,000 distinct genes (Powell, 2013; Roy, 2005). Some were turned on (upregulated), while others were turned off (downregulated), most notably those affecting wound healing, immunity, cardiovascular function, sleep and metabolism.

In another study (Dusek, 2008), researchers examined how mind-body practices eliciting a relaxation response affected genetic transcriptional profiles. Regular practitioners were compared to novices (with eight-week relaxation training) and healthy controls. Results showed 2,209 genes were differently expressed in regular practitioners compared to controls, and 1,561 genes were differently expressed in novices compared to controls. Regular practitioners and novices shared 433 differently expressed genes, and the genes involved affected cellular metabolism, oxidative phosphorylation and response to oxidative stress. The authors postulated that the relaxation response might have long-term beneficial effects on gene expression as it relates to oxidative and psychological stress.

The importance of stress in the expression of variant genotypes is also not to be underestimated. For example, despite ideal SNP coding for genes TCF7L2 and IRS1, increased cortisol will triple the release of insulin to carbohydrates such as grains, starches, sweets and fruits, forcing the body to treat one apple as the equivalent of three apples, or one cookie as a whole box!

In one study (Park, 2016) looking at the association of the variant MC4R C-allele with obesity, once adjusted for other variables, the results indicated that those individuals with high stress levels had a stronger association with higher BMI and preferential intake of processed and fat-dense foods over fruits and vegetables. The authors concluded that the interaction of stress and the variant allele of MC4R altered energy intake and eating behaviour to an extent that exceeded that of the variant allele alone.

In another study (De Oliveira, 2011) looking at the combined effect of diet and the stress hormone cortisol on adiponectin production, rats were fed either a normal or high-fat diet for 12 weeks. As expected, the high-fat group demonstrated increased blood sugar levels and a fourfold reduction in ADIPOQ gene expression. The rats then underwent surgery, removing their adrenal glands to decrease serum cortisol levels. Half the rats had the cortisol replaced with injections while the other half got saline. The rats that had their cortisol replaced continued to show high levels of blood glucose and insulin along with reduced levels of circulating adiponectin. ADIPOQ gene expression in fat, liver and muscle tissue was up to seven times lower than normal. The rats that got saline, and therefore on-going low cortisol, normalized their glucose and insulin and increased their adipose tissue ADIPOQ expression fourfold. Persistent high cortisol levels present in chronic stress can be expected to have a similar effect on adiponectin, glucose and insulin even with a relatively healthy diet.

There are a variety of different genes involved in the stress pathway. Some genes are directly responsible for the production of stress hormones (cortisol, adrenalin and noradrenalin) or their releasing factors (CRH from the hypothalamus and ACTH from the pituitary gland). Other genes control enzymes and pathways involved in metabolizing these hormones or neurotransmitters, or code for receptors that bind them.

Variance in the SNP coding for certain genes leads to over- or underactivity of the sympathetic nervous system and stress pathways.

These genes have the potential to impact the production of stress hormones that can then alter the functioning and expression of many other genes, as well as increase the adverse effects that stress has on metabolism, food breakdown and energy storage. They will also affect levels of anxiety, quality of sleep, healing and immunity.

Two approaches are therefore required to address the impact of stress. First, as stress itself influences gene expression, controlling the level of stress in your life is vital. This is achieved using a number of approaches including lifestyle changes, diet and supplementation. Second, by looking at your coding for a number of stress-associated SNPs, we can identify and treat any increased genetic risk for overactivity within the stress pathway (HPA axis).

We will look at four important stress-related genes and their relevant SNPs:

- ADRB2
- NR3C2
- CRHR1
- FKBP5

ADRB2 SNP rs1042714
Beta-2 Adrenergic Receptor SNP (Q27E Gln27Glu)
Normal/Ancestral allele – C
Variant/Risk allele – G

The ADRB2 gene codes for the Beta-2 ADrenergic Receptor, one of the receptors that mediates the effect of catecholamines (epinephrine/norepinephrine) on cellular function and metabolism. The B2 receptor binds epinephrine with 30 times greater affinity than norepinephrine and is a major receptor promoting lipolysis (fat breakdown) on human adipose cells.

Genes affecting the regulation of catecholamine function are thought to be important in the development of obesity through their effect on energy expenditure, lipolysis and fatty acid metabolism. A number of

SNPs affecting adrenergic receptors have been identified and linked to obesity in a number of populations. ADRA2A is associated with higher BMI, percentage of body fat and insulin resistance. The ADRB2 rs1042713 SNP has been linked to insulin resistance and hyperlipidemia but not obesity.

The ADRB2 SNP rs1042714 has one of the clearest associations with obesity, with one research paper (Large, 1997) demonstrating a Relative Risk of 7 and an Odds Ratio of 10 in the population studied. The variant allele was found to be twice as common in obese subjects (Odds Ratio 2.14) and those with type 2 diabetes (Odds Ratio 2.13) in a Japanese population (Ishiyama-Shigemoto, 1999). As the β2-adrenergic receptor (ADRB2) is involved in energy balance regulation through the stimulation of both thermogenesis and lipid mobilization from adipose tissue, variant expression in this gene has the potential to have a profound effect on weight gain and adiposity.

G-allele
- Increased BMI and obesity risk
- Increased risk of insulin resistance and type 2 diabetes
- Increased risk of hyperlipidemia
- Increased sensitivity to carbohydrates
- Slower metabolic rate
- More at risk from a sedentary lifestyle
- Respond well to dietary changes
- Increased blood pressure
- Increased production of inflammatory cytokines TNF and IL10 (A cytokine is a substance secreted by immune cells that stimulates other immune responses, such as inflammation, in this case an increase in TNF and IL10.)
- Altered leptin production and thus increased food cravings and slower metabolism
- Decreased thermogenesis

Research shows that this SNP interacts with diet to significantly impact body weight. G-allele individuals will gain more weight on a regular diet but will also *lose* more weight if they adopt a calorie-reduced diet. In a 12-week controlled weight loss study (Ruiz, 2012), obese women followed a low-energy mixed diet (55% carbohydrates, 30% lipids and 15% proteins) providing 600 kilocalories less than individually estimated energy requirements based on resting metabolic rate (RMR). Researchers found a significant interaction between the ADRB2 GG polymorphisms and diet-induced changes on body weight. Women carrying the G-allele had greater reduction in body weight than did C-allele carriers. Interestingly, the G-allele was associated with a greater reduction in lean mass, indicating that simple calorie restriction may not be the healthiest option in this genotype. Other studies have found weaker association between the rs1042714 SNP and dietary-induced weight loss. Exercise appears to be an important modifying factor for this SNP. In one study, the G-allele was associated with higher BMI in those with a sedentary lifestyle but not in those that were active.

And in one further example of gene–nutrient interaction, the rs1042714 SNP is found to be linked to obesity in individuals consuming a high-carbohydrate diet with an Odds Ratio of 2.56 (Martinez, 2003).

NR3C2 SNP rs5522
Nuclear Receptor Subfamily 3 group (MRI180V, ile180val)
Normal/Ancestral allele – A
Variant/Risk allele – G

The NR3C2 gene codes for the mineralocorticoid receptor (MR). Besides being important in the control of sodium in the body, it is also an important determinant of the body's response to stress. It belongs to the nuclear receptor superfamily and functions as a transcription factor mediating the effects of aldosterone on a variety of target tissues, including the distal parts of the nephron, the distal colon, the cardiovascular and central nervous systems, and brown adipose tissue. MR possesses the same affinity for glucocorticoids (including cortisol) as for mineralocorticoids. In the kidney, the effect of cortisol on the MR is minimal due to the coexistence of a neutralizing enzyme.

However, in the brain, the effect is significant, particularly as the MRs are concentrated in the limbic system including the hippocampus and hypothalamus. It is proposed that the MR exerts a controlling effect on the stress pathway (HPA axis) both in the resting state and under conditions of acute stress.

Note: *The nomenclature for this SNP is somewhat confusing in the literature. Although always referred to as rs5522, the allele description is inconsistent. In the standard format, A is given as the normal or reference allele, and G as the risk or variant allele. Most research papers studying the MR SNP use this terminology as does* SNPedia. *Some sources, including 23andMe, refer to the inverse strand and "flip" the bases such that A (normal) becomes T, and G (risk) becomes C. (See DNA Strand Terminology page 29 and SNP Nomenclature and Orientation page 40)*

We will use the generally accepted terminology (Normal – A, Risk – G). So if your 23andMe coding is T, then use A in this section. If your 23andMe coding is C, then use G.

G-allele
- Reduced MR expression and activation
- Decreased binding and response to cortisol
- Impaired HPA axis feedback
- Greater and more prolonged response to stress
- Poor stress resilience
- Increased anxiety/depression risk
- Increased blood pressure risk
- Increased food cravings and eating disorders

The main impact of the risk allele (G) is reduced feedback within the HPA axis. The stress response is designed to be beneficial and short-acting—think escaping from the tiger. However, when prolonged, stress causes numerous detrimental metabolic and health effects. Under normal circumstances, cortisol released from the adrenal glands circulates back to the brain and hypothalamus to switch off the stress pathway (HPA axis). In the presence of chronic stress, the development of cortisol resistance leads to impaired negative feedback from peripherally produced cortisol, resulting in persistent activity within the HPA pathway. The G-allele imparts similar cortisol resistance through its effect on MR structure and function.

Studies show that the cortisol and heart-rate responses to acute psychosocial stress are profoundly increased in G-allele carriers and that resilience to stress in these individuals is impaired (DeRijk, 2005). They have an enhanced level of chronic perceived stress, that is, mental stress that is not truly threatening but is treated by the body in the same way, for example, a work deadline or being stuck in traffic. This may have lasting effects, with some studies showing limbic dysfunction and heightened risk of psychological disorder in those exposed to chronic or repetitive stress as a child or adult. Learning is impaired and the response to reward-activated behaviour altered even in psychologically normal subjects.

There is an association between the G-allele with both ADHD (Attention Deficit Hyperactivity Disorder) and the severity and expression of eating disorders related to self-perception and body perfectionism.

CRHR1 SNP rs242939
Corticotropin Releasing Hormone Receptor
Normal/Ancestral allele – T
Variant/Risk allele – C
Note: SPedia *references the minus strand so A is normal and G is variant.*

The CRHR1 gene encodes a receptor that binds neuropeptides of the Corticotropin Releasing Hormone (CRH) family. CRH is a major regulator of the hypothalamic-pituitary-adrenal (HPA) pathway that mediates our response to stress. This receptor protein is essential for the activation of pathways that regulate numerous physiological processes including endocrine and autonomic responses to stress, reproduction, immune response and obesity. It is present in both the central and peripheral nervous system. Within the brain, it is particularly found in the limbic system, hypothalamus and pituitary gland. Upregulation (increased number) of receptors in the pituitary gland is associated with increased anxiety and risk of panic disorder. Upregulation within the limbic system affects feedback and results in hypersensitivity to stress and cortisol levels that remain persistently high following a stressful stimulus. Due to the extensive influence of CRH on both psychological and metabolic wellbeing, CRHR1-blocking drugs are being investigated for their potential role in the treatment of depression, anxiety, eating disorders and addiction as well as metabolic disorders such as obesity and metabolic syndrome.

A number of polymorphisms associated with this gene have been identified and have a significant impact on both the stress response itself and its long-term implications. The rs242938 SNP variant A-allele is associated with a heightened stress response and increased alcohol intake following stress exposure in adolescents. The rs242939 variant C-allele is associated with increased risk of depression and an altered response to antidepressants.

As with other stress genes, polymorphisms that affect functioning, sensitivity and feedback within the HPA axis have the potential to augment the deleterious effects stress has on the body and in particular weight and metabolism.

C-allele
- Increased CRH expression
- Increased stimulation of the HPA axis
- Loss of negative feedback
- Hypersensitive stress response and persistent activation
- Increased risk of eating disorders

FKBP5 SNPs rs3800373 and rs1360780
FK506 Binding Protein

FK506 Binding Protein 5 (FKBP5) is a key molecule in the stress response. It has a profound regulatory effect on the glucocorticoid receptor (GR), controlling binding, activation and transcriptional processes associated with the receptor protein.

A number of polymorphisms have been found to affect this binding protein and subsequently alter activity and feedback within the stress response pathway with subsequent wide-reaching effects. Two of the most important are rs3800373 and rs1360780.

The minor alleles in both SNPs are associated with increased expression of FKBP5, altered feedback in the HPA axis, impaired cortisol recovery following stress and higher self-reported anxiety. This is caused by the allele itself and from epigenetic alteration in DNA methylation at this gene locus. There is reduced binding of miRNA (micro-RNA) in the translation process, resulting in an increase in overall FKBP5 expression.

Individuals with the risk alleles have increased risk of adult PTSD if they have been exposed to childhood trauma. Individuals with variant alleles for FKBP5 demonstrate altered functioning in the frontotemporal-parietal network on functional MRI, which may underpin the impaired interpretation of stressful events and the increased sensitivity within the HPA axis. FKBP5 expression is markedly increased following glucocorticoid exposure in the limbic system of the brain, particularly the amygdala and PVN, while the hippocampus shows persistent high baseline FKBP5 levels. Variations in FKBP5 glucocorticoid responsiveness are implicated in dysfunctional feedback in the HPA axis, and conditions associated with this disorder including PTSD, anxiety and major depressive disorder (MDD).

FKBP5 appears to play a significant role in energy homeostasis. FKBP5 overexpression leads to obesity and impaired glucose tolerance in animal models. The rs1360780 risk allele is associated with reduced ability to lose weight. Individuals with risk alleles that lead to higher levels of FKBP5 will have increased cortisol activity during fasting and diets that mimic fasting as these conditions lead to HPA axis activation. This overactivity will have an adverse effect, preventing weight loss and possibly promoting weight gain.

FKBP5 rs3800373
Normal/Ancestral – C (Risk allele)
Variant allele – A

Note: *There is some inconsistency with the reporting of alleles for rs3800373. Much of this stems from confusing "normal" with "minor." It appears that for this SNP, the normal (reference or ancestral) allele is the minor allele as it has a lower frequency (33%) than the variant allele (67%). The normal allele is also the "risk" allele. The emergence of the variant as the more beneficial allele might be because it confers an evolutionary advantage.*

C is therefore the normal allele, and A is the variant. As with other SNPs, the complementary nucleotide is often reported such that G is normal, and T is variant.

FKBP5 has been studied in individuals with chronic musculoskeletal pain. Individuals carrying the minor allele have an increased risk of developing a post-traumatic pain syndrome. In a recent study of 1,500 individuals who had experienced motor vehicle trauma, those homozygous for the risk allele (C) had significantly higher pain levels. This effect was markedly amplified if the individual reported high levels of stress following the accident.

FKBP5 rs1360780
Normal/Ancestral allele – C
Variant/Risk allele – T

Individuals with the T-allele have twice the risk of cortisol hyper-reactivity compared to normal individuals. In a study of patients undergoing bariatric surgery for obesity, those with the T-allele stopped losing weight earlier in the post-operative period than those with the C-allele. They also demonstrated substantially lower overall weight loss than normal individuals.

Risk alleles for both **rs3800373 and rs1360780** are associated with:

- Increased FKBP5 expression
- Impaired HPA axis feedback
- Increased cortisol activity
- Enhanced stress response
- Obesity risk with impaired weight loss ability
- Poor response to fasting
- Increased risk of PTSD and MDD
- Increased risk of chronic post-traumatic pain syndrome

THE METABOLIC EFFECTS OF STRESS

With regards to metabolism, cortisol acts to increase blood sugar levels by releasing stores from the liver and muscle. This is to help prepare the body for the increased energy expenditure associated with resolving the fight-or-flight situation. While this may be beneficial when escaping from a marauding tiger, it is not needed when sitting in traffic or at our desk, times when our modern perceived stress hits. Without immediate exercise, the rise in blood sugar is profound. In response to this, the pancreas produces insulin, our storage hormone that acts to sweep the sugar out of the blood, storing it primarily as fat. The associated cortisol results in this deposition being mainly in the central abdominal area of the body.

Cortisol also has a profound effect on our appetite. Prolonged exposure promotes increased food intake and cravings for sweets and carbohydrates. It is responsible for the "midnight munchies" that propel you to the fridge in the early hours of the morning!

Insulin levels naturally rise as we age, for example, you'll secrete more insulin in response to a bagel at 50 years old than you did at 20. In addition, the rise in blood sugar caused by persistent cortisol promotes further insulin secretion. Over time, the recurrent stimulation of insulin release leads to insulin resistance, a relative insensitivity of the tissues in the body to this hormone. The result is higher and more prolonged peaks of insulin production and eventually a number of metabolic abnormalities associated with weight gain such as diabetes, high blood pressure and heart disease.

One of the most detrimental and profound effects of chronic stress is weight gain. In a society where 65% of individuals are overweight and 31% are clinically obese, chronic stimulation of the HPA axis can therefore be viewed as one of the most prevalent risk factors to our health. Cortisol inhibits the release of leptin. This hormone simulates α-MSH and inhibits neuropeptide-Y, reducing our appetite after a meal and "jump-starting" our metabolism. The inhibition of leptin not only increases food cravings but reduces our metabolic rate and impairs fat burning by over 60%. Stress also triples the release of insulin in response to grains, starches, sweets and fruits, forcing the body to treat one slice of bread as if it were three, one cookie as three cookies and so on. This promotes amplified fat storage, particularly in the abdominal region where white fat cells have three times the number of cortisol receptors on their surface. To make matters worse, CRH and cortisol block the production and binding of both serotonin and dopamine. This combination of imbalanced hormones destabilizes mood and stimulates further food cravings. Cortisol also inhibits PGC1-α, a substrate that is produced in our muscles when we exercise. PGC1-α increases the production of irisin, the hormone that converts white inflammatory fat into brown thermogenic fat. By blocking this pathway, cortisol promotes weight gain, blood sugar instability and diabetes, independent of diet and exercise.

Individuals with any of the risk alleles for stress genes need to be cognizant of their tendency to express the adverse effects of chronic stress including carbohydrate sensitivity, increased visceral fat storage, enhanced food cravings and poor satiety response. Maintaining a lower calorie diet will help offset the effects of reduced thermogenesis. Individuals also need to maintain healthy muscle mass (particularly if carrying the ADRB2 G-allele), which means adequate protein intake.

STRESS GENES TREATMENT

DIET

Specific dietary recommendations are based on your other genes, but in general, if you have more than one of the stress gene risk alleles:

- Be conscientious and adhere closely to your genetic carbohydrate recommendations
- Avoid processed foods, which increase cravings
- Ensure you achieve the gene-recommended protein intake to stabilize blood sugars
- Having referenced your other genes, reduce your daily calorie intake by 200 to 300 calories per day
- Try to only have a maximum of one cup of coffee per day. If you consume more than three cups a day, change your cups of coffee to half-caffeinated and half-decaffeinated, still consuming the same number of coffees a day. Slowly cut back by one cup every three days.

EXERCISE

There is ample evidence to support the role of exercise in stress management. Its effects are mediated through a number of physiologic and psychological mechanisms. Regular aerobic exercise is associated with:

- Lower sympathetic nervous system and HPA axis activity
- Increased levels of serotonin in the brain
- Increased levels of endogenous opioid such as endorphins
- Increased brain-derived neurotrophic factor (BDNF)
- Improved neural remodelling within the limbic system
- Desensitization to anxiety-associated symptoms such as rapid heart rate
- Increased self-awareness and self-efficacy
- Distraction

Recommendation: Two to two-and-a-half hours of moderate- to high-intensity exercise per week. Increase to three to four hours if carrying the ADRB2 G-allele

PHYSICAL THERAPIES (BODY WORK)

- One hour of therapeutic body work each week, such as massage, reflexology or shiatsu. This may be any type of bodywork, but it must be a type that is performed on you, not one that you do on your own.

RELAXATION TECHNIQUES

- One hour of relaxation, such as yoga or meditation, per week. This may be done at home with a video, at a gym in a class, or with a personal trainer. This may be split into two 30-minute sessions per week.
- 10 minutes of deep breathing each day. Do not worry if your mind travels at first when you start breathing. Simply refocus your thoughts towards your breath and continue. As you progress, you will find it easier to stay focused.
- Take a 20-minute bath with lavender oil two times a week.

SUPPLEMENTS

- Serenetin Plus. Use this table to gauge your Sereniten Plus dose. For each SNP, identify whether you have a risk allele. Count them up and refer to the dosage guideline below.

GENE	ALLELE	
	NORMAL	RISK
ADRB2	C	G
NR3C2	A	G
CRHR1	T	C
FKBP5	A	C

- For one risk allele, take one Sereniten Plus twice a day on an empty stomach for eight weeks, then reduce to one per day.
- For two risk alleles, take two Sereniten Plus twice a day on an empty stomach for eight weeks, then reduce to one per day.
- For three or four risk alleles, take two Sereniten Plus twice a day on an empty stomach for 12 weeks, then reduce to one per day.
- Take additional Sereniten Plus, as needed, for stressful days, and take one in the middle of the night if waking frequently.

Sereniten Plus

Sereniten Plus is a combination of casein decapeptide (Lactium®), L-theanine and vitamin D to support the hypothalamic-pituitary-adrenal (HPA) axis and feedback. It is used for stress support, cortisol regulation and weight management. Lactium® and L-theanine have been shown to provide a calming effect and may support normal sleep that is affected by stress.

Lactium® is a bioactive decapeptide alpha-1 sequence, isolated from milk. It is effective at restoring normal HPA function and feedback. Lactium® works at three areas of the HPA axis:

- *Lactium® binds specifically to the BZD site of the GABA-A receptor and does not bind to the PBR site of the GABA-A1 receptor responsible for the sedating effects seen with benzodiazepines.*
- *Lactium® increases the sensitivity of the hypothalamus to cortisol, re-establishing receptor sensitivity feedback within the HPA axis. It reduces the amount of CRH produced in response to stress.*
- *Lactium® decreases the amount of cortisol released by the adrenal glands during acute and chronic stress.*

NOTE: *Although derived from milk, due to the small size of the molecule, Lactium® bypasses the immune system and does not induce an allergic response. It is therefore tolerated by those with dairy or lactose sensitivity or allergy.*

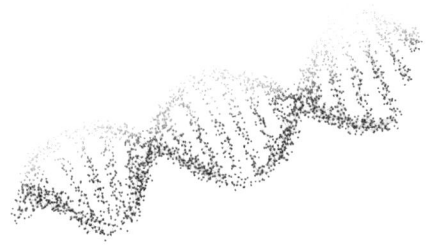

CHAPTER 18
Case Study #5
Stress and Diet

Donna is 48-year-old female who had gained 21 pounds over the past year despite her usual healthy diet of protein and vegetables, moderate fats, and little to no simple carbohydrates. She had even tried to "clean up" her diet by cutting out all sugars and reducing alcohol to one glass of wine per week. She reported having food cravings for sweets and fats, and these cravings worsened whenever she "cheated" with cheese or chocolate. Cravings were rare but intense and something she really wasn't accustomed to. Interestingly, she did notice that the food cravings decreased when she ate fewer calories and resisted the cravings.

Nine months prior to the onset of her weight gain, she had gone through a divorce and started a new job at the same time. Her normal sleep pattern changed such that she was waking most nights between 2 a.m. and 4 a.m. (a classic high-cortisol sign) with racing thoughts that prevented her from falling back asleep until just before her alarm clock went off. She reported feeling severely stressed during that time, but now the divorce was over and she was more comfortable in her new job, she didn't understand why she still had disrupted sleep and feelings of anxiety.

Donna's genetic profile included the following coding:

- ADIPOQ rs17366568 – AA: lower adiponectin, better with caloric restriction
- TCF7L2 – CT: moderate sensitivity to carbohydrates and moderate insulin response
- IRS1 – TT: normal glucose and insulin response to carbohydrates
- APOA2 – CC: increased LDL, weight and inflammation with more than 22 grams of saturated fat
- FTO – AA: increased leptin resistance, lower adiponectin and increased ghrelin, increased cravings for energy-dense foods such as fats and sweets
- NR3C2 – GG: cortisol resistance, impaired HPA feedback, prolonged stress response.
- CRHR1 – CT: increased CRH and HPA axis stimulation

Donna was already eating a diet very close to her genetic ideal, which is why she had always been slim in the past. However, the stress leading up to and going through the divorce, along with starting a new job, caused her sensitive NR3C2 and CRHR1 genes to stimulate her stress pathways to such a degree that they turned on her FTO, ADIPOQ and APOA2 genes. These genes together altered the production of adiponectin, leptin and ghrelin, slowing the metabolic rate, encouraging fat storage and greatly increasing food cravings. Her stress gene coding (NR3C2 and CRHR1) meant she had less ability to switch off her stress response and revert back to the "quiet side" (parasympathetic) of her nervous system. The production of stress hormones remained high and continued to disrupt her sleep and stimulate her metabolic and dietary genes.

Based on her genetics, I recommended the following protocol:

- Tri-Metabolic Control: two capsules 30 minutes before lunch and dinner every week for eight weeks and then one out of every four weeks

- Sereniten Plus*: two capsules twice a day on an empty stomach, and one capsule as needed in the middle of the night when waking between 2 a.m. and 4 a.m. After eight weeks, reduce to one capsule twice a day.
- Melatonin PR: three milligrams before bedtime
- Daily guided meditation
- Regular exercise including yoga and one bodywork treatment (such as a massage) every four to six weeks
- PureLean Fiber: one scoop with fattier meals or, if needed, in-between meals to control cravings
- Intermittent fasting: 16 hours fasting (see Chapter 20). No change in quantity or proportion of food but a change only in meal timing

Results
- One week later she had significantly fewer food cravings in the evening as a result of the TMC and Sereniten Plus.
- She began waking more rested within five days and was sleeping through the night by two weeks as a result of the Sereniten Plus and melatonin.
- Two weeks later she lost four-and-a-half pounds with no real change in diet or exercise.
- Two months later she had lost 18 pounds.
- One year later she had lost 28 pounds and was comfortable maintaining this weight.

*Sereniten Plus is a combination of casein decapeptide (Lactium®), L-theanine and vitamin D to support the hypothalamic-pituitary-adrenal (HPA) axis and feedback. It is used for stress support, cortisol regulation and weight management. For more information, see Appendix 2.

This case study demonstrates the importance of epigenetics, that is, the role of external factors such as diet and stress in the expression of genes that affect metabolism. Addressing this issue is key to the effectiveness and permanence of any treatment protocol.

I do not want to see a three-month "quick fix" followed by a rapid return to old habits and a rebound of weight. In Donna's case, once the stress and metabolic hormones were reset with the Sereniten Plus and Tri-Metabolic Control along with lifestyle changes and intermittent fasting, the expression of the poorly functioning metabolic genes was "turned off," allowing her to lose weight and feel healthier. Once she was stable, I suggested she consider intermittent fasting on a more regular basis given her FTO AA coding and cycle the supplements in and out every four weeks in order to maintain optimum gene function.

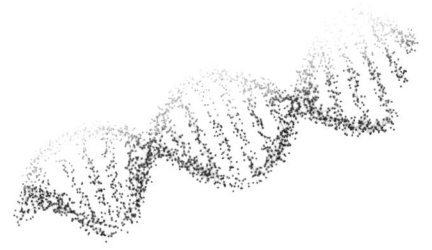

CHAPTER 19
Proteins, Fats and Carbohydrates
Which Genes Influence Your Ideal Balance of Macronutrients

> *Note: For more details on the gene SNPs included in this section, please refer to their individual chapters.*

Adjusting the nutrient content of your diet according to your genes is essential in order to maximize your health, reduce your risk of metabolic disorders and control your weight. As you have seen in previous chapters, numerous SNPs impact your ability to handle proteins, fats and carbohydrates. Putting it all together in order to create an effective dietary plan can be difficult, so this chapter aims to give you some simple genetic guidelines to use when deciding how to balance the three macronutrients protein, fat and carbohydrate. However, while the important macronutrient SNPs are discussed in this chapter, the influence of others—including metabolic SNPs (MC4R, PPARG and ADIPOQ) along with the stress gene SNPs—is essential to consider when planning dietary balance. In addition, it should be noted that in my practice and within *GeneRx.ca*, I use more extensive and complex algorithms incorporating other SNPs not included in this book.

I often incorporate an eight-week "genetic retraining" period during which dietary changes are more stringent. This is discussed more extensively within individual SNP chapters along with recommendations on exercise and supplements, which often play a key role in treatment.

Proteins

Proteins are complex molecules comprised of chains of amino acids, smaller organic molecules that form the building blocks of each protein. The body uses 20 amino acids to form proteins, and while able to manufacture many of them, nine are considered "essential." These essential amino acids are histidine, isoleucine, leucine, lysine, methionine, phenylalanine, threonine, tryptophan and valine and have to be obtained from the food we eat.

Proteins are essential to the body for the manufacture of tissues, hormones, antibodies and innumerable structural elements— everything from a muscle fibre to a skin cell, the hemoglobin that transports oxygen in your blood, the enzymes that digest your food and the insulin that controls your blood sugar. All are one of the estimated 10,000 proteins that create the structure of your body and allow it to function.

As a fuel source, proteins provide similar energy density to carbohydrates (four kilocalories or 17 kilojoules per gram) but are used preferentially for their amino acid content. As the body cannot store "spare" amino acids, dietary intake is needed to provide the material necessary to maintain its structural and functional integrity and allow the rebuilding of proteins such as muscle that are continually being degraded. As part of a balanced diet, protein is also important as it slows down the absorption of carbohydrate from the gut, helping control blood sugar levels and insulin release.

Recommendations for the amount of protein we need varies greatly. Values from 0.6 grams per kilogram (g/kg) of body weight per day (5.5 grams per 20 pounds) to 1.7 g/kg body weight per day (15.5 grams per 20 pounds) are suggested dependent on age, activity level and need to build muscle. However, most current research indicates we eat way too much protein in general, and this leads to inflammation and fat storage. As the body is unable to store amino acids, excess is either excreted by the kidneys or converted to sugar or fat. While a small amount of this may be used as fuel, the majority is stored, leading to potential weight gain. High levels of dietary protein can cause dehydration, gout, liver and kidney damage, and calcium loss. Even more concerning is research by Levine (2014), who found that individuals aged 50 to 65 years of age, consuming 20% or more of their calories from animal protein sources, had a 75% higher mortality risk and were four times more likely to die from cancer than those consuming a low-protein diet (less than 10% of calories from protein). However, this does not seem to hold true if the protein source is plant-based (Giovannucci, 2016).

The quality of protein we ingest appears to be extremely important. Diets high in red meat have been shown to increase the risk of heart disease, diabetes, cancer and obesity in a number of studies, and although this was initially attributed to the saturated fat content, this assumption is now questionable. Red meat that is processed or charred appears to be much more harmful, indicating that it's the chemical composition rather than the fat content that imposes risk. Individuals eating red meat on a regular basis have up to three times higher levels of the metabolite trimethylamine N-oxide (TMAO) than those eating white meat, fish or vegetable protein. TMAO is produced in the gut by bacteria during digestion and is linked to increased heart disease risk.

The protein sources I recommend contain highly digestible and bioavailable amino acids including the essential ones with low or zero saturated fat content (for a more complete list, see Appendix 1):

- Fish
- Egg whites
- White meat (chicken or turkey)

- Whey protein isolate (Whey Satisfied by Douglas Laboratories)
- Hydrolyzed beef protein with collagen (PurePaleo by Designs for Health)

Calculating Your Protein Portion

Your protein intake is primarily determined by your FTO gene coding and is modified according to activity level. Here's how to calculate how much protein you should consumer per meal:

Step 1: Look at your FTO gene coding: AA (variant); TA or TT (normal)

Step 2: Assess your activity level:
- Inactive: less than 30 minutes of exercise twice a week
- Average: 30 to 45 minutes of exercise three times a week
- Active: 45 minutes to two hours of exercise three or more times a week

Step 3: Refer to Table 2 to calculate your daily protein requirement
- Multiply the number in the table by your bodyweight (kilograms or pounds)
- Divide by three to give the amount of protein per meal. This number stays the same for each meal even if you are only eating twice a day, such as during intermittent fasting.

Example: The table gives a value of 1 g per kg bodyweight (0.45 g per pound) and you weigh 60 kg (132 pounds). Total protein per day is 60 grams/3 = average 20 grams per meal. 20 grams of protein would be three ounces of chicken, five or six egg whites or 2/3 cup of 0% fat plain Greek yogurt. **See protein food tables in Appendix 1 for more examples.**

Table 1: Daily protein requirements based on FTO coding and activity level

	FTO AA	FTO TA	FTO TT
Inactive	1g/kg (0.45g/lb)	0.8g/kg (0.36g/lb)	0.6g/kg (0.27g/lb)
Average (Exercise 2 or 3 times a week)	1.1g/kg (0.5g/lb)	0.9g/kg (0.41g/lb)	0.7g/kg (0.32g/lb)
Active (Daily exercise)	1.2g/kg (0.54g/lb)	1g/kg (0.45g/lb)	0.8g/kg (0.36g/lb)

Note: A useful way to gauge how much protein there is in a protein source is to use the size of your hand:
1. Measure and learn the size of your hand (see picture below).
2. Use the chart to estimate the physical size of a protein source that would contain the number of grams you need in a meal.
3. Use your hand as a guide when estimating protein content.

Example:
- Your hand measures 7 centimetres x 16 centimetres (depth is assumed to be 1 centimetre)
- You need 20 g of protein at a meal
- Your protein source is chicken
- 20 g chicken is approximately 5 centimetres x 10 centimetres
- You need a piece of chicken about 1/2 the size of your hand

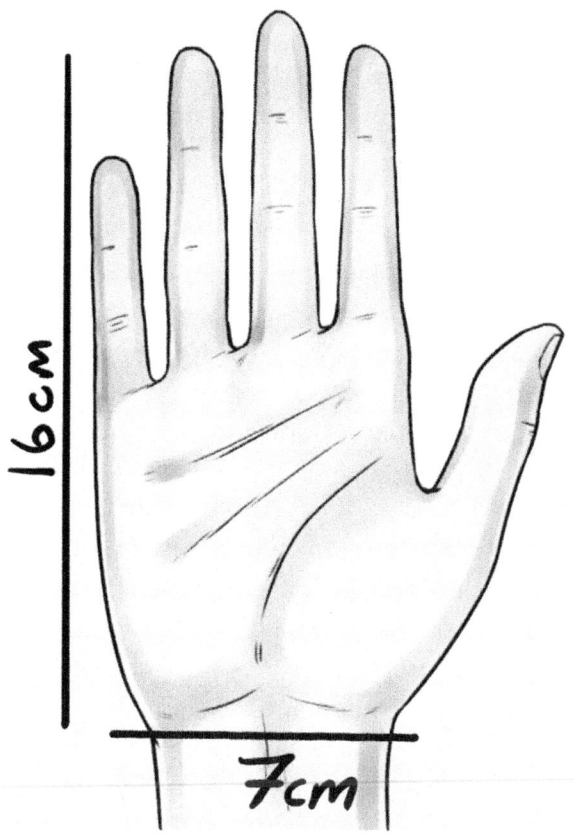

Figure 2: Calculating your hand size

Table 2: Examples of protein source size (See Appendix 1 for full table.)

	Chicken	Fish	Red Meat
15 g	4 x 10 x 1 cm	7 x 10 x 1 cm	4 x 10 x 1 cm
20 g	5 x 10 x 1 cm	9 x 10 x 1 cm	5 x 10 x 1 cm
25 g	6 x 14 cm	11 x 10 x 1 cm	6 x 10 x 1 cm
30 g	8 x 10 x 1 cm	14 x 10 x 1 cm	8 x 10 x 1 cm

Fats

Fats are an essential macronutrient for our body. They are our most important fuel source, providing 80 to 90% of our energy during rest or normal daily activity. One gram of fat provides over twice as much energy (nine calories per gram) as carbohydrate or protein (four calories per gram). They are also vital for endurance sports as our carbohydrate stores alone only last 90 to 120 minutes. Fats are used to construct and support the membrane of every cell in our body. They are used as precursor chemicals in the manufacture of many hormones and are essential for the absorption of the fat-soluble vitamins A, D, E and K. Stored fats provide insulation and cushioning and improve the integrity of skin, hair and nails.

Dietary fats are divided into four types—all of which have different properties—with classification based on their structure. Each fat molecule is made up of one glycerol unit and three fatty acids, hence, the other term for fat, *tri*glyceride. The fatty acid building blocks are classified according to the number of carbon atoms and the number of double bonds between those carbon atoms. Medium-chain fatty acids, for example, have tails of six to 12 carbon atoms, while long-chain ones have 13 to 21. Fatty acids with chains that contain no double carbon bonds are termed **saturated** fats and are usually solid at room temperature. Those with at least one double bond are termed **unsaturated**. If there is just one, they are termed **monounsaturated** while those containing multiple double bonds are **polyunsaturated**. Most often these are liquid at room temperature. Unsaturated fats have a chemical structure that can be *cis* or *trans*, with trans-fats being predominantly man-made and associated with poorer health implications. Whereas the body can manufacture many of its required fats from basic building blocks, there are two **essential** fats that must come from our diet. These are the omega-3 and omega-6 fatty acids; the three or six number refers to where the first double bond is located on the carbon chain. The three types of omega-3 fatty acids are alpha-linoleic acid (ALA), eicosapentaenoic acid (EPA) and docosahexaenoic (DHA). The body needs ALA in the diet and can use it to manufacture

EPA and DHA. The main type of omega-6 is linoleic acid, which is required in our diet.

While omega-3 fatty acids are generally considered anti-inflammatory and omega-6 fatty acids as pro-inflammatory, both are required for optimum functioning of the immune system. Unfortunately, a preponderance of omega-6 has a deleterious effect on health, and this has profound implications in a society where the average diet has a ratio of omega-6 to omega-3 of about ten-to-one. The ideal ratio is about two-to-one and possibly closer to one-to-one.

The body has a tremendous ability to store fat in adipose cells. This was originally an evolutionary advantage, protecting the individual against starvation in times of famine. Fatty acids are key for energy production (ATP production). When compared to other macronutrients such as carbohydrates or proteins, fatty acids yield the most ATP on an energy per gram basis. This is why fatty acids are the foremost storage form of fuel in humans, animals and, to a lesser extent, plants. Unfortunately, we now live in a society where there is often unlimited food, and this protective mechanism has backfired, leading to excess fat accumulation.

The role of fat in health and disease has been the subject of discussion and controversy for many years. In the late 1970s and early 1980s, the "low-fat" diet craze took off, fuelled by two studies that linked obesity and disease risk to fat intake. What was not made clear was type of fat, saturated or unsaturated, at a time where general knowledge of nutrition amongst the public was rudimentary at best. The result was a generation that grew up avoiding fat and defaulting to carbohydrates for calories. Unfortunately, the excess carbohydrates promoted even greater weight gain along with increased type 2 diabetes, high cholesterol and metabolic syndrome.

The realization that "low-fat" wasn't working led to the "low-carb" craze, championed by Atkins and now popular in keto-type diets in which fats replaced carbohydrates as a source of energy. Unlike the

Atkins diet, in which gradual reintroduction of complex carbohydrates is allowed, a keto diet promotes permanent restriction of all carbohydrate sources and forces the body into a state of starvation-like ketosis. Such diets have been buoyed by studies indicating that heart disease is more related to inflammation than dietary fat and that certain diets such as the Mediterranean Diet that incorporate a higher percentage of saturated and unsaturated fats reduce heart disease risk. Keto diets have shown benefit in the control of epilepsy, blood sugar control in diabetes and liver function, with conflicting research on how harmful it is to the kidneys. Certainly, many people lose weight, but the long-term effects are unknown, particularly as the fat choices people make may not be that healthy. While choosing unsaturated over saturated fats may be recommended, in reality this can be hard to do. The health risks of long-term, high-saturated-fat intake remain unknown, but from what we know about genetics, this may prove detrimental.

The pendulum has truly swung from carbohydrate to fat, and while diet trends come and go according to research, using our genetics can give us some individual guidelines that help us make a more rational decision on intake. I am not a proponent of one particular diet but prefer to use genetic information to recommend intake levels of proteins, carbohydrates and *saturated fats* rather than all fats.

The major genes that dictate fat consumption, particularly saturated fats, are APOA2, FABP2 and FTO. FTO homozygote variant (AA) carriers, for example, weigh an average three kilograms (6.6 pounds) more than do TT individuals and have 1.67 times the risk of obesity compared to TT individuals. This rises to 2.5 times if ingesting a high-carbohydrate or high-fat diet. APOA2 individuals with the CC genotype have been shown in multiple populations to be at a significantly increased risk of obesity compared to CT or TT individuals when they ingest more than 22 grams of saturated fat per day. And for FABP2, a study in the journal *Metabolism* (Chamberlain, 2009) found that AAs or GAs that ate a diet containing 53 grams or more of saturated fat per day had lower HDL-to-total cholesterol ratios; higher cholesterol,

LDLs and triglycerides; and higher levels of insulin resistance. The integration of these genes' SNPs is important, as looking at them individually can give conflicting information. This is why my *GeneRx.ca* program considers multiple SNPs when making recommendations. Overall, from my clinical experience, I find APOA2 to be the most important with regards to saturated fat, and this is reflected in my treatment protocol, as follows:

APOA2
- If you are variant for APOA2 (CC), you need to stick to less than 22 grams of saturated fat per day
- If you are heterozygote for APOA2 (CT), you need to stick to less than 28 grams of saturated fat per day
- If you are normal for APOA2 (TT), you do not have a limit on saturated fats; however, it is still not wise to consume them in excess

FTO
- If you are variant for FTO (AA), you need to stick to less than 30 grams of saturated fat per day. This reduces to less than 22 grams per day if you are variant (CC) for APOA2.
- If you are heterozygote for FTO (TA), you need to stick to less than 35 to 38 grams of saturated fat per day unless variant for APOA2 (CC); then you need to reduce saturated fats to less than 22 grams per day.
- If you are normal for FTO (TT), you do not have a limit on saturated fats unless you are variant for APOA2 (CC); then you need to reduce saturated fats to less than 22 grams per day.

FABP2
- If you are variant for FABP2 (AA), you need to stick to less than 53 grams of saturated fat per day. This reduces to less than 30 grams of saturated fat per day if you are variant for FTO (AA) and a further reduction to 22 grams per day if you are variant (CC) for APOA2.

- If you are heterozygote for FABP2 (GA), you need to stick to less than 53 to 60 grams of saturated fat per day. This reduces to less than 30 grams of saturated fat per day if you are variant for FTO (AA) and a further reduction to 22 grams per day if you are variant (CC) for APOA2.
- If you are normal for FABP2 (GG), you do not have a limit on saturated fats. This reduces to less than 30 grams of saturated fat per day if you are variant for FTO (AA) and a further reduction to 22 grams per day if you are variant (CC) for APOA2.

Table 3: SNP integration table for saturated fat intake

		FTO			FABP2		
		AA	TA	TT	AA	GA	GG
APOA2	CC	<22g/day	<22g/day	<22g/day	<22g/day	<22g/day	<22g/day
	TC	<28g/day	<28g/day	<28g/day	<28g/day	<28g/day	<28g/day
	TT	<30g/day	35-38g/day	No Limit	<53g/day*	53-60g/day *	No Limit *

*Unless
FTO is AA then <30g/day
FTO is TA then 35-38g/day

For more information on foods high or low in saturated fat, please see Appendix 1 Food Tables and the sidebars on pages 103 and 140.

Carbohydrates

The third macronutrient is carbohydrate. Used primarily as a fuel source, carbohydrates also form a part of important molecules such as DNA and structural components of cell membranes. Carbohydrates comprise the sugars, starches and fibres (cellulose) found in grains, fruits, vegetables, legumes, dairy products and alcohol. Chemically they contain carbon, hydrogen and oxygen, forming a saccharide or sugar molecule. They vary in size from the basic simple sugar monosaccharides such as glucose and fructose to long, complex, indigestible plant fibres such as cellulose. Monosaccharides are strung together in chains to form polysaccharides. The shortest of these has just two sugar units (disaccharides) and include sucrose (plants) and lactose (dairy), while longer chains include starches found in vegetables, glycogen (our body's storage form of sugar) and insoluble fibre.

Nutritionally, carbohydrates are divided into simple and complex, also termed high glycemic and low glycemic, reflecting how they are handled by digestion, absorption and metabolism. Simple carbohydrates include the mono- and disaccharides found in sweets, deserts and fruits, while complex carbs occur in legumes, vegetables and nuts. When we eat simple carbohydrates, they are either absorbed immediately (glucose) or rapidly broken down and absorbed. This leads to a swift rise in blood sugar levels and a corresponding increase in insulin. Complex carbs are broken down and absorbed more slowly, leading to a more gradual rise in blood sugar and insulin. While grains of all types contain complex carbs, the refined versions (such as white flour and white rice) have their fibre and protein removed such that their breakdown and absorption is faster when compared to the unrefined versions.

Under the influence of insulin the body has tremendous ability to store carbohydrates. Absorbed sugars are converted to glycogen stores in muscle and liver cells and, following transformation to fatty acids, to fat stores in adipose and other tissues.

The role of simple dietary carbohydrates in the development of disease is well established. There is ample evidence to support the role of excess sugars in the development of type 2 diabetes, independent of body weight. Hyperinsulinemia, metabolic syndrome and dyslipidemia accompany this risk. In terms of weight gain and obesity, there is evidence that high simple sugar intake including that contained in sweetened soft drinks is a significant contributor to the epidemic. The carbohydrate-insulin model (CIM) of obesity links the hormonal changes that lead to insulin resistance and diabetes to excess weight gain. However, studies have failed to demonstrate a clear and simple link between overall carbohydrate intake and obesity.

> **Choosing the Right Carbohydrate**
>
> *Try to avoid simple, high-glycemic carbohydrates including sugars and sweets. Note that fruit is considered a simple (high-glycemic) carbohydrate despite the fact it contains some fibre. Fruit juice is worse than the fruit itself. To put that in perspective, one apple weighing 233 grams has 31 grams of carbs with 23 grams of sugar. One standard size KitKat bar has 27 grams of carb and 21 grams of sugar. Yes, the apple has more sugar and carb than the KitKat chocolate bar! The best types of fruit to choose are berries. Some of the complex carbs such as broccoli, cauliflower and mushroom contain a better ratio of fibre to sugar. For example, ½ cup of broccoli has 5.5 grams of total carb, with only 1.1 gram of sugar and 2.5 grams of fibre. But ½ cup of brown rice has 22.4 grams of carb, 21.9 of that being sugar.*
>
> *Generally speaking, the "good carbs" that you want to fill your plate with are vegetables and salads, the foods with colour. These foods can essentially be consumed in unlimited quantity. Vegetables that are excluded from the "unlimited" category are the starches such as potato, sweet potato, yam, squash and pumpkin. While still considered complex (low-glycemic), they are not as good a choice as other sources. When choosing grains, use unrefined versions such as brown rice or whole-wheat flour.*

Researchers are quick to point out that available studies have significant limitations in terms of populations examined and variability of dietary carbohydrate ingested. There is certainly evidence that refined sugars and grains are more harmful, and this, along with the balance of simple to complex carbohydrates, likely has a substantial impact. Genetics also plays a major role and may explain at least some of the inconsistencies within and between populations.

Two of the more important genes I look at when considering carbohydrate intake are TCF7L2 and IRS1. Look at your coding for both genes and then the recommendations below. You should follow the diet indicated by your highest risk coding for either gene. For example, if you code TT for TCF7L2 and CT for IRS1, then follow the TCF7L2 diet recommendations. If your coding is of equal risk for each gene, then follow either program but make sure to check your Gene Interactions.

	TCF7L2	IRS1
Highest Risk	TT	CC
Medium Risk	TC	CT
Lowest Risk)	CC	TT

TCF7L2
Normal allele – C
Risk allele – T

The T-allele of TCF7L2 is strongly linked to the development of type 2 diabetes across multiple populations. Numerous studies have demonstrated the SNP increases population-attributable risk by 16 to 21%. Heterozygous individuals have a Relative Risk of 1.45 while the homozygous genotype confers a Relative Risk of 2.41. Adherence to a Mediterranean Diet (high unsaturated fats and complex carbohydrates) has been shown to markedly reduce fasting glucose and lipids in TT carriers. A diet high in simple sugars is correlated with increased expression of the TT genotype while high fibre intake to reduce its influence.

Treating TCF7L2 **TT**

DIET – first eight weeks

- Avoid simple carbohydrates at two of the three meals per day

- Simple carbohydrates can be eaten at one meal per day but limit the amount to ½ the physical size of the protein for that meal. Simple carbohydrates include grains (breads, pastas, rice, corn, popcorn, legumes, quinoa, etc.), starches (potato, sweet potato, yam, squash, etc.), sweets, fruits or alcohol.
- Complex vegetable carbohydrates can be eaten in unlimited quantities at all meals
- Lower saturated fats in the diet to less than 30 to 35 grams per day

DIET – after 8 weeks

- Avoid simple carbohydrates at one of the three meals per day
- Simple carbohydrates can be eaten at two meals per day but limit the amount to ½ the physical size of the protein for that meal. Simple carbohydrates include grains (breads, pastas, rice, corn, popcorn, legumes, quinoa, etc.), starches (potato, sweet potato, yam, squash, etc.), sweets, fruits or alcohol.
- Complex vegetable carbohydrates can be eaten in unlimited quantities at all meals
- Lower saturated fats in the diet to less than 30 to 35 grams per day

Treating TCF7L2 **CT**

DIET – first eight weeks

- Avoid simple carbohydrates at one of the three meals per day
- Simple carbohydrates can be eaten at two meals per day but limit the amount to ½ the physical size of the protein for that meal. Simple carbohydrates include grains (breads, pastas, rice, corn, popcorn, legumes, quinoa, etc.), starches (potato, sweet potato, yam, squash, etc.), sweets, fruits or alcohol.

- Complex vegetable carbohydrates can be eaten in unlimited quantities at all meals
- Lower saturated fats in the diet to less than 30 to 35 grams per day

DIET – after 8 weeks

- Simple carbohydrates can be eaten at three meals per day but limit the amount to ½ the physical size of the protein for that meal. Simple carbohydrates include grains (breads, pastas, rice, corn, popcorn, legumes, quinoa, etc.), starches (potato, sweet potato, yam, squash, etc.), sweets, fruits or alcohol.
- Complex vegetable carbohydrates can be eaten in unlimited quantities at all meals
- Lower saturated fats in the diet to less than 30 to 35 grams per day

Treating TCF7L2 **CC**
- No specific carbohydrate restrictions, but a diet higher in complex carbohydrates is recommended for overall health

---

Gene Interactions

Look at IRS1 and FTO to further assess carbohydrate intake:

- *If you code variant CC for IRS1 and/or variant AA for FTO, then it becomes even more important that you adhere to the above guidelines for TCF7L2*

Look at APOA2 to further assess your saturated fat intake:

- *If you are homozygote variant CC for APOA2, then your saturated fat content needs to be reduced to 22 grams per day*
- *If you are heterozygote TC for APOA2, then your saturated fat content needs to be reduced to 28 grams per day*

IRS1
Normal allele – T
Risk allele – C

Numerous polymorphisms in the IRS1 gene are associated with type 2 diabetes and susceptibility to insulin resistance. Along with other SNPs at the same IRS1 gene locus, the rs2943641 variant (C) allele is associated with an increased ratio of visceral to subcutaneous fat, insulin resistance, metabolic syndrome, poor lipid profile, increased risk of type 2 diabetes and coronary artery disease.

Treating IRS1 CC

Diet – first eight weeks

- Avoid simple carbohydrates at two of the three meals per day
- Simple carbohydrates can be eaten at one meal per day but limit the amount to ½ the physical size of the protein for that meal. Simple carbohydrates include grains (breads, pastas, rice, corn, popcorn, legumes, quinoa, etc.), starches (potato, sweet potato, yam, squash, etc.), sweets, fruits or alcohol.
- Complex vegetable carbohydrates can be eaten in unlimited quantities at all meals
- Keep saturated fats below 28 grams per day

Diet – after 8 weeks

- Avoid simple carbohydrates at one of the three meals per day
- Simple carbohydrates can be eaten at two meals per day but limit the amount to ½ the physical size of the protein for that meal. Simple carbohydrates include grains (breads, pastas, rice, corn, popcorn, legumes, quinoa, etc.), starches (potato, sweet potato, yam, squash, etc.), sweets, fruits or alcohol.
- Complex vegetable carbohydrates can be eaten in unlimited quantities at all meals
- Keep saturated fats below 28 grams per day

Treating IRS1 *TC*

Diet – first eight weeks

- Avoid simple carbohydrates at one of the three meals per day
- Simple carbohydrates can be eaten at two meals per day but limit the amount to ½ the physical size of the protein for that meal. Simple carbohydrates include grains (breads, pastas, rice, corn, popcorn, legumes, quinoa, etc.), starches (potato, sweet potato, yam, squash, etc.), sweets, fruits or alcohol.
- Complex vegetable carbohydrates can be eaten in unlimited quantities at all meals
- Keep saturated fats below 28 grams per day

Diet – after 8 weeks

- Simple carbohydrates can be eaten at three meals per day but limit the amount to ½ the physical size of the protein for that meal. Simple carbohydrates include grains (breads, pastas, rice, corn, popcorn, legumes, quinoa, etc.), starches (potato, sweet potato, yam, squash, etc.), sweets, fruits or alcohol.
- Complex vegetable carbohydrates can be eaten in unlimited quantities at all meals
- Keep saturated fats below 28 grams per day

Treating IRS1 *TT*

- Although this coding means you have a lower risk of insulin resistance, type 2 diabetes and metabolic syndrome, there is evidence that this effect is reduced if your diet has a high total fat or saturated fat-to-carbohydrate ratio. Therefore, I recommend keeping your saturated fat below 30 to 35 grams per day and avoid fat-dense diets such as keto.
- Although carbohydrates are not limited, I recommend sticking to low-glycemic complex sources to maximize the benefit of your coding

- Women with TT can increase their fat intake a little (about 35 to 40 grams per day) *unless* contraindicated by APOA2 and FTO
- Men can increase their carbohydrate intake a little unless variant for TCF7L2

Gene Interactions

Look at TCF7L2 and FTO to further assess carbohydrate intake:

- *If you code variant TT for TCF7L2 and/or variant AA for FTO, then it becomes even more important that you adhere to the above guidelines for IRS1*
- *Keep saturated fats below 22 grams per day if variant (C) for APOA2*

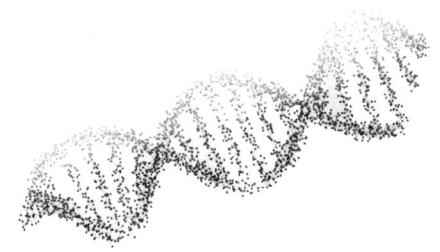

CHAPTER 20
Meal Timing and Intermittent Fasting
Which Genes Influence when You Should Eat

The timing and number of meals in a day is just as important as their dietary content, and much like the pendulum for fats and carbohydrates, opinions as to what regimen is best have swung significantly over the past few years. Recommendations have varied from the traditional three meals a day through frequent snacking of six to eight meals to the two meals a day of intermittent fasting (I.F.).

Theories concerning meal timing are often based on what we know about how the body handles the food we eat. They consider digestion, absorption and metabolism and examine the hormonal response to food and the factors affecting hunger and satiety. Unfortunately, this information changes over time as new research becomes available, and this now includes the influence of genetic coding.

Note: Before making any changes to calorie intake or meal timing, individuals with established diabetes (types 1 or 2), particularly if using insulin, should always consult with their health-care practitioner.

Snacking and Frequent Small Meals

The myth that frequent small meals were the key to weight loss likely arose from two sources. The first involved dietary studies performed in the late 1990s that showed how frequent small carbohydrate meals could lead to more stable blood sugar and insulin levels along with lower cholesterol. Aimed primarily at diabetics, the concept spread rapidly to normal and then overweight individuals. The second related to research indicating that metabolic rate increased temporarily after a meal. This led to the concept that more meals would somehow "supercharge" the body and allow it to burn off fat. However, that was the '90s. Ideas have changed as new research has become available. In addition, the fact that our population is growing steadily larger and unhealthier is certainly a compelling argument against frequent small meals being a dietary panacea!

In order to dispel the myth of frequent small meal eating, consider some of the theories proposed as to why it works. For example, does it really "supercharge" our metabolism? The answer is "no." While it is true that there is a temporary increase in the metabolic rate associated with the ingestion, absorption and metabolism of food, it only amounts to about 10% of your calorie intake and is independent of meal size. So whether you eat three meals of 900 calories or six meals of 450 calories (both totalling 2,700 calories), you will only increase your metabolism by 270 calories per day. Unfortunately, the frequent small meal option reduces your leptin levels, which actually lowers your metabolic rate!

Eating numerous small carbohydrate meals during the day may well lead to more stable blood sugar, but at what cost? The persistent secretion of insulin this type of diet causes will actually increase the risk of insulin resistance and metabolic syndrome. The studies that showed how frequent small meals could reduce cholesterol only compared small carbohydrate meals to large carbohydrate meals rather than to balanced protein-complex carbohydrate intake. This latter type of diet achieves stable blood sugars without overstressing the pancreas and also stops the liver from producing cholesterol.

For those on a diet, frequent small meals are offered as the answer to food cravings and satiety. That is a little like trying to get someone to stop smoking while allowing them to light up every time they have a nicotine yearning! Recent research on the real reasons behind hunger and craving relate to neurochemical changes in the brain, abnormal behaviour patterns that need to be changed not reinforced.

Probably the biggest problem with the whole concept of frequent small meals is that they rapidly become frequent large meals. Research shows that having a snack between meals does not reduce the size of the next meal. In addition, the availability of fast, unhealthy food means that snacks often become highly calorific themselves. Giving an individual carte blanche to eat whenever they like in a society where food is so readily available may be a popular and painless option, but it is highly unlikely to be successful in the long term. It will certainly never address the many health issues associated with overeating and a dysfunctional metabolism.

Normal human physiology is not designed for frequent small meals and remains essentially unchanged from that of our prehistoric ancestors. Neanderthal man was more accustomed to starvation and long gaps between meals than tucking into limitless dinosaur snacks by the fire. As such, humans are hardwired to be hungry and to store food away as fat. The two major hormones insulin and leptin work together to manage fat stores. After a meal, insulin rises for three hours, initially replacing glycogen stores and then shunting any extra calories into fat. As insulin levels fall, we become able to access our fat stores as a source of energy. Eating another meal or snack at this point causes a further release of insulin, which not only inhibits our ability to burn fat but also acts as a strain on the pancreas. This secondary rise in insulin is more prolonged and, when the cycle is repeated, will eventually lead to hyperinsulinemia and insulin resistance, forerunners of metabolic syndrome. This pattern additionally leads to leptin resistance resulting in food cravings and a slower metabolism.

An important question is whether these guidelines should be changed in the athletic individual. Current research argues against the concept of "carb-loading" before exercise but does favour adequate dietary intake to support daily training and recovery by restoring glycogen levels. If the interval between training periods is short (eight to 16 hours), then increasing meal frequency will be necessary to achieve adequate intake. However, for the majority of individuals with at least a 24-hour interval between training periods, three balanced protein-carbohydrate meals per day provides the healthiest option.

Meal timing in the elite or high-level endurance athlete is a matter of preference. Some individuals may be able to eat a large meal one or two hours before training, whereas others may need a series of smaller, easily digested meals. Increased hydration with each meal is essential but content should generally be balanced. The exceptions include intake during exercise, which should be predominantly carbohydrate, and post-exercise meals for individuals training or competing later the same day. In these athletes, early post-exercise carbohydrate intake has been shown to promote faster glycogen synthesis and better endurance recovery.

Fasting

The traditional three-meals-a-day routine allows for about five hours between meals and a longer period (eight to 10 hours) overnight. Immediately following a meal, you enter a "fed state," which means your body is digesting and absorbing the nutrients you have eaten. This generally lasts about three to five hours and is associated with high insulin levels that control blood sugar levels by promoting its storage as glycogen and fat. Absorbed fats are also stored as triglycerides in adipose tissue. The body uses the available sugar as fuel and preserves your fat stores.

After three to five hours, you enter a "post-absorptive" or "early fasting" state during which blood sugar levels are no longer maintained by the food absorbed from the GI tract. As blood sugar levels fall, the body switches off insulin and increases glucagon production, which promotes the release of glucose from its stored form—glycogen in the liver, thereby maintaining blood sugar levels. Glucagon also causes fat cells to begin to break down triglycerides to release fatty acids that provide an additional source of fuel.

As the fasting state continues, the body enters a "prolonged fasting" state with further changes to metabolism. A well-fed individual has enough energy stores for one to three months but only enough carbohydrate (glycogen) for about 12 to 36 hours. Therefore, as glycogen stores become depleted, the body needs to replace them by using glycerol from mobilized fat stores and amino acids from muscle protein.

As fasting progresses towards what is essentially a starvation state, the body switches its fuel source from glucose to fatty acids and ketone bodies (of "keto-diet" fame). It does this to preserve protein and the structural integrity of tissues. Muscle switches to fatty acids as a source of fuel early on because glucagon prevents it from utilizing blood glucose. After about three days, the liver begins to produce large amounts of ketone bodies, molecules produced by the incomplete metabolism of fatty acids. The kidney acts to preserve these valuable ketone bodies, which would otherwise be excreted in large amounts in the urine. The liver does continue to produce glucose as a minimum blood level is required for the brain and red blood cells, but the amount is diminished. The ketone bodies it produces now act as an alternate fuel source for the brain, heart and other tissues. Initially forming about one third of fuel requirements, by three weeks starvation, ketone bodies become the major fuel source, greatly protecting protein stores (muscle). Early in starvation, muscle breakdown can be as high as 75 grams per day, while later this is reduced to 20 grams per day by the use of ketone bodies. There is evidence that the switch to ketone metabolism is, in part, responsible for some of the beneficial effects of intermittent fasting (I.F.), and this has driven the "keto" movement as keto diets aim to mimic starvation without the calorie restriction.

Calorie-restriction diets lead to weight loss and improvements in metabolic markers in most studies but have proved hard for individuals to maintain. Diets that promote I.F. rely on achieving the "metabolic switch" from glycogen and glucose utilization to fatty acids and ketones. Once the switch has been "flipped," the body has moved entirely from fat storage and synthesis to fat breakdown (lipolysis) and metabolism. These diets therefore have the potential to not only promote weight loss and combat obesity but also address metabolic disease such as type 2 diabetes.

There is extensive research into the benefits of I.F. including:
- Weight loss: partially a result of reduced overall calories and somewhat impaired if calories are increased at two meals to compensate for the missed meal. Weight loss is also a result of changes to metabolism including increased metabolic rate and a switch to ketone energy use
- Lower insulin levels, higher growth hormone and adiponectin: promotes fat burning and improves muscle building
- Improves insulin resistance: reduces the risk of type 2 diabetes and may reverse it. There is also a reduced risk of metabolic syndrome
- Increased longevity in animal species tested: possibly a result of improved mitochondrial efficiency and reduced level of reactive oxygen species (free radicals) known to promote inflammation
- Reduced overall levels of inflammation with improvements in conditions such as arthritis
- Reduced cardiovascular risk factors: lower blood pressure and improved lipid profile
- Improved cellular health: increased autophagy, which is a cellular clean-up process that may slow aging and reduce cancer risk
- Cancer: *animal* studies show reduced cancer risk
- Brain function and repair: *animal* studies show improved brain cell metabolism, decreased oxidation, better healing potential and reduced risk of neurodegenerative disorders. Alzheimer's disease symptoms were improved in one small human study on the effects of I.F.

Epigenetic Effects of I.F.

- Muscle: improved fatty acid oxidation, response to stress and resistance to oxidative damage
- SIRT1: increased expression reduces tissue response to stress, which includes apoptosis (cell death). This may slow aging and reduce cancer risk. SIRT1 expression in adipose tissue improves fat mobilization and energy balance. Via stimulation of PPARG expression, it stimulates thermogenesis.
- Increased expression of leptin (LEP) and adiponectin (ADIPOQ) genes through altered methylation of DNA

However, much of the research thus far is on animals, and whether this translates into human benefits remains to be seen. In addition, there are likely population differences concerning I.F. For example, one study showing impaired glucose tolerance in women compared to men following a period of I.F.

Many of the ill effects of fasting relate to prolonged fasting in which there is nutrient deficiency including lack of vitamins and minerals. This is less of an issue with the short-term programs discussed here, but individuals need to be cognizant of their micronutrient intake. Problems such as fatigue, poor concentration and nausea are mostly temporary but can persist in some individuals. There is some evidence that I.F. leads to increased stress and cortisol and this will result in impaired blood sugar regulation. However, it is likely that the chronic stress and cortisol issue is a result of HPA axis (stress response pathway) dysfunction rather than an I.F. issue. After all, from an evolutionary perspective, fasting for 12 to 16 hours is probably the norm and should be well tolerated by our primitive physiology. As discussed in other areas of this book, addressing chronic stress and altered cortisol feedback is an essential part of the function of your metabolic genes.

> ### Types of Intermittent Fasting (I.F.)
>
> - *Calorie Restriction (CR)* – an ongoing reduction in caloric intake without malnutrition
> - *Intermittent Fasting (I.F.)* – fasting for 12 to 16 hours on a daily basis
> - *Time-Restricted Feeding (TRF)* – eating only within a specific eight- to 12-hour period of the day
> - *Alternate-Day Fasting (ADF)* – no calories are consumed on fasting days with unrestricted food intake on "feast" days
> - *Alternate-Day Modified Fasting (ADMF)* – similar to TRF but with 25% of the baseline energy needed on "fasting" days alternated with unrestricted food intake on "feast" days
> - *Periodic Fasting (PF)* – fasting only one or two days a week and consuming unrestricted food on five or six days per week
> - *Fasting Mimicking Diet (FMD)* – this five-day fasting pattern involves lowering caloric intake to 700 calories per day, with a significant reduction in protein and sugars, and no saturated fats to mimic a fasting response in the body. The five-day fast is completed once every three months.

Genetic Coding and Meal Timing

As with any other type of diet, your metabolic SNP coding can help identify whether you are a candidate for I.F. As we have seen above, meal restriction can have significant benefits, but overall results, ease of participation and side effects may vary between individuals. For my patients, I use the following guidelines:

My I.F. Regimen
- Two meals per day with one small snack in between **only if needed**
- All food to be consumed within an eight-hour period
- 16 hours fasting
- During fasting, you can have fluids including coffee and tea (which can contain a small amount of milk but no sugar). Avoid sugary drinks and fruit juice.
- Meal content (protein, fat and carbohydrate) according to your dietary SNPs

I use certain gene SNPs to determine if I.F. is your best diet option or whether it is a possibility if you wish to try it. There are only two genotype situations in which I do not recommend it, both because it offers no real benefit and because of the likelihood it will be poorly tolerated. Those are FTO TT and MC4R TT.

FTO and MC4R are the principle SNPs I use to determine your suitability for I.F. If you code poorly for either of these genes, then I recommend I.F. as your best form of food intake, certainly for the first eight weeks during the genetic retraining period.

I recommend I.F. for:
- FTO – AA and TA
- MC4R – CC and TC

If you are MC4R TT, then you do not need I.F. but it is not contraindicated if you wish to try such a diet.

ADIPOQ is the other gene I use to advise on I.F. If you code poorly, then I recommend I.F. as a diet option, but it is not essential.

I suggest I.F. for:
- ADIPOQ rs17366568 - AA and GA
- ADIPOQ rs17300539 - GG and AG

For normal coding (rs17300539 AA and rs17366569 GG), I.F. is not contraindicated if you wish to try it.

FTO and PPARG

For individuals that have healthy coding for FTO (TT) and PPARG (GG), I generally recommend against I.F. I find that patients with such coding tolerate this form of diet poorly and gain no significant metabolic benefit.

Table 4: Intermittent Fasting (I.F.) recommendations

	SNP			
	FTO	MC4R	ADIPOQ rs17366568	ADIPOQ rs17300539
Coding	AA | TA | TT	CC | CT | TT	AA | GA | GG	GG | AG | AA
Definite I.F.	X | X |	X | X |	| |	| |
I.F. Recommended	| |	| |	X | X |	X | X |
I.F. Possible	| |	| |	| | X	| | X
Not Indicated	| | X	| | X	| |	| |

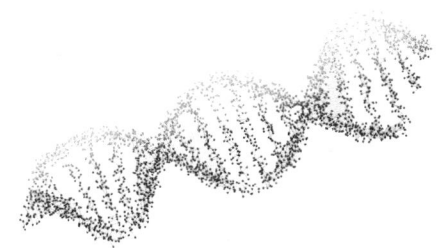

CHAPTER 21
Case Study #6
Meal Timing and Intermittent Fasting

Susan is a generally healthy 48-year-old, perimenopausal woman. She came to see me because over the past six to nine months she had gained 27 pounds in unwanted weight without any changes to her diet or exercise program. She had never previously been persistently overweight but was prone to gaining five pounds or so during times of stress. In addition, during the past year, she had had difficulties sleeping, waking both at 2 a.m. and 4 a.m. She had tried pharmaceutical and natural sleeping pills and had been started on hormone replacement treatment by her GP, but nothing seemed to work. She would fall asleep easily but woke repeatedly during the night. In the morning, she would feel tired and unrested and would have low energy throughout the day. Overall, she reported her mood being low.

In an attempt to lose the weight, she had stopped eating all sugars, starchy grains and most fruits and sweets, but it had not helped. She was eating a higher amount of protein, an abundance of green vegetables, good unsaturated fats in moderation and quite low saturated fats.

Susan's genetic profile included the following coding:

- TCF7L2 – CC: normal insulin response to carbohydrates
- IRS1 – TC: slight increase in insulin to carbohydrates
- GIPR* – CC: normal insulin response and GI inflammation with carbohydrates
- FTO AA: slower metabolism, increased risk of obesity, leptin resistance, low adiponectin and increased ghrelin. Intermittent Fasting recommended
- MC4R – TC: increased cravings and emotional overeating. Intermittent Fasting recommended
- NR3C2 – GG: cortisol resistance, impaired HPA feedback, prolonged stress response.

This SNP is not included in the book but is a part of my workup in this case.

Susan had always kept her slower metabolism and metabolic hormonal imbalance in check through a clean and balanced diet. It wasn't until perimenopause, when the production and release of her stress hormones increased and her estrogen decreased, that she began to notice changes.

The MC4R C-allele resulted in decreased levels of satiety, causing more frequent eating and snacking, especially with foods high in saturated fat. It also led to emotional overeating and low mood.

The rise in cortisol and falling estrogen triggered her FTO and MC4R expression, so although her diet remained balanced and fairly good for her genes, the extra sensitivity meant she needed to become a little stricter, particularly in terms of meal timing.

Based on her genetics, I recommended the following protocol:

- Intermittent fasting
    - Two meals per day with one small snack in between **only if needed**

- All food to be consumed within an eight-hour period
- 16 hours fasting
- Low-calorie diet: 800 to 1,100 calories per day
- Tri-Metabolic Control. Two capsules twice a day 30 minutes to one hour before her two meals for one month to help reset all three metabolic hormones that were disrupted when FTO and MC4R expression increased, and to reset those genes.
- Sereniten Plus. Two capsules twice a day on an empty stomach, one dose before bed until she was sleeping fully every night for two weeks in a row. Then reduce the dose to one capsule twice a day.

Within two weeks, Susan had already lost seven pounds. She was only waking once at night and would fall back asleep fairly quickly. Four weeks later she had lost 12 pounds, was feeling strong and healthy, was sleeping through the night and felt her mood improve during the day. At this point, she dropped the Tri-Metabolic Control. By five months she had lost 32 pounds, was still sleeping well and felt fully rested on waking every day. Two years later, her weight remains stable and her sleep pattern consistently restful. She increases the Sereniten Plus as needed if she experiences a period of increased stress. This keeps her NR3C2 gene balanced and avoids triggering MC4R.

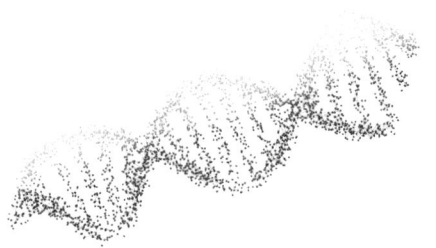

CHAPTER 22
Conclusion

Over the past ten years, analysis of personal genetics has become a key component in my Naturopathic Medicine practise. It has helped me address individual health issues, solve difficult clinical problems and provide truly personal and focussed care for my patients. Diets, exercise programs, lifestyle changes and supplement regimens are not "one size fits all" options and it takes knowledge of someone's DNA blueprint to formulate a protocol that suits them best. Patients that have struggled for years to manage their weight, energy and overall health, finally understand what is going on within their body. Genetic analysis enables them to make sense of their idiosyncrasies and choose a path that is both manageable and effective. They return telling me they feel the best they have in years.

John Naisbitt wrote, "We are drowning in information but starved for knowledge." (Naisbitt, 1982). That statement is even truer today. Information such as your DNA coding is easily accessible, with millions of individuals ordering commercially available tests every year. Yet for most people, the results provide little opportunity to improve their knowledge of how best to live their lives. The ream of information received is often overwhelming, making it hard to identify SNPs that are important or relevant. Trying to use the data to discover more about your health, diet or metabolism is even more difficult. My hope is that this book has allowed you to understand what your genetic analysis means and how it can be used to identify your personal strengths and weaknesses. I have focussed on the important areas of diet, metabolism and weight using SNPs that find most significant when treating my patients. SNPs that not only have a profound impact on many aspects of your health, but also offer opportunities for intervention should you have at-risk coding. Armed with this knowledge you can start to make the changes that will allow you to optimize your diet, health and weight. To fix your genes and fit your jeans!

The field of personal genetic testing is rapidly expanding, with new SNPs and new health associations being discovered all the time. It is exciting to finally see health being addressed on a truly individual basis. However, sometimes the music can be lost in the background noise. Having read this book I believe you will have the knowledge you need to tune your hearing and follow your own personal DNA melody.

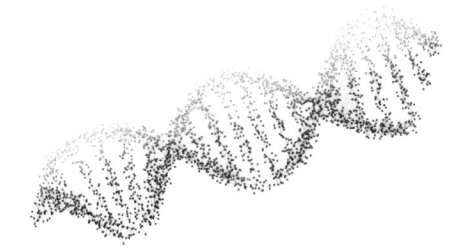

APPENDIX 1
Food Tables
A Simple Guide to Food Portions

Table 1: Fat content for different protein sources
I recommend choosing protein sources with the lowest Saturated Fat per 100 grams

Protein Source	Protein per 100 Grams (3.5 oz)	Fat per 100 Grams (3.5 oz)	Saturated Fat per 100 grams (3.5 oz)
Egg Whites	11 grams	0 grams	0 grams
Whole Egg	13 grams	11 grams	3.3 grams
Salmon (Atlantic)	24 grams	13 grams	3 grams
Salmon (Coho)	24 grams	3.5 grams	1 gram
Light Tuna (in water)	24 grams	0.6 grams	0 grams
Trout	21 grams	6 grams	1.4 grams
Cod	20 grams	0.6 grams	0 grams
Chicken (skinless breast)	32 grams	3.6 grams	1 gram
Turkey (skinless breast)	30 grams	7 grams	2 grams
Veal	24 grams	8 grams	3 grams
Pork	21 grams	30 grams	11 grams
Beef (lean)	32 grams	11 grams	4.5 grams
Firm Tofu (low fat)	16 grams	8 grams	1 gram
Whey Satisfied Protein	60 grams	0 grams	0 grams
Cottage Cheese (1% fat)	12.6 grams	2.5 grams	1.5 grams
Greek Yogurt (0% fat)	10 grams	0 grams	0 grams
Regular Yogurt (2% Fat)	3.5 grams	1.6 grams	1 gram
PurePaleo Protein	78 grams	1 gram	0.5 grams

Protein Portion Sizes

Once you know how many grams of protein you need at a meal (see Chapter 19), the tables on the following pages will help you calculate how much of each protein source you need to eat. For example, if your calculation indicates you require 15 grams of protein at a meal, you should eat four egg whites or 60 grams of salmon. (I recommend choosing protein sources with the lowest Saturated Fat content.)

Table 2: Portion size for 15 grams of protein

Protein Source	Portion Size (Grams/Ounces)	Portion Size (Dimensions)	Saturated Fat
Egg Whites	140 g/5 oz	4 egg whites	N/A
Whole Egg	115 g/4 oz	3 whole eggs	4.6 grams
Salmon (Atlantic)	60 g/2.2 oz	6cm x 10cm x 1cm	1.8 grams
Salmon (Coho)	60 g/2.2 oz	6cm x 10cm x 1cm	0.6 grams
Light Tuna (in water)	60 g/4 ooz	6cm x 10cm x 1cm	0 grams
Trout	70 g/2.5 oz	7cm x 10cm x 1cm	1 gram
Cod	75 g/2.6 oz	7cm x 10cm x 1cm	0 grams
Chicken (skinless breast)	50 g/1.75 oz	4cm x 10cm x 1cm	0.47 gram
Turkey (skinless breast)	50 g/1.75 oz	4cm x 10cm x 1cm	1 gram
Veal	60 g/4 oz	5cm x 10cm x 1cm	1.8 grams
Pork	70 g/2.5 oz	6cm x 10cm x 1cm	7.7 grams
Beef (lean)	45 g/1.6 oz	4cm x 10cm x 1cm	2 grams
Firm Tofu (low fat)	180 g/6.4 oz	1 cup	1.3 grams
Whey Satisfied Protein	25 g/0.9 oz	1 ½ scoops	0 grams
Cottage Cheese (1% fat)	120 g/4.2 oz	½ cup	1.8 grams
Greek Yogurt (0% fat)	150 g/5.3 oz	½ cup	0 grams
Regular Yogurt (2% Fat)	400 g/14 oz	1 ⅔ cups	1 gram
PurePaleo Protein	19 g/0.7 oz	¾ scoop	0.1 gram

Table 3: Portion size for 20 grams of protein

Protein Source	Portion Size (Grams/Ounces)	Portion Size (Dimensions)	Saturated Fat
Egg Whites	190 g/6.7 oz	5 egg whites	N/A
Whole Egg	150 g/5.3 oz	4 whole eggs	6 grams
Salmon (Atlantic)	80 g/2.8 oz	8cm x 10cm x 1cm	2.4 grams
Salmon (Coho)	80 g/2.8 oz	8cm x 10cm x 1cm	0.8 grams
Light Tuna (in water)	80 g/2.8 oz	8cm x 10cm x 1cm	0 grams
Trout	90 g/3.2 oz	9cm x 10cm x 1cm	1.3 gram
Cod	100g/3.5 oz	9cm x 10cm x 1cm	0 grams
Chicken (skinless breast)	62 g/2.2 oz	5cm x 10cm x 1cm	0.63 gram
Turkey (skinless breast)	67 g/2.3 oz	5cm x 10cm x 1cm	1.3 grams
Veal	80 g/2.8 oz	7cm x 10cm x 1cm	2.4 grams
Pork	93 g/3.2 oz	8cm x 10cm x 1cm	10.3 grams
Beef (lean)	63 g/2.2 oz	5cm x 10cm x 1cm	3 grams
Firm Tofu (low fat)	240 g/8.5 oz	1⅓ cup	1.7 grams
Whey Satisfied Protein	33 g/1.2 oz	2 scoops	0 grams
Cottage Cheese (1% fat)	160 g/5.6 oz	¾ cup	2.4 grams
Greek Yogurt (0% fat)	200 g/7 oz	¾ cup	0 grams
Regular Yogurt (2% Fat)	500 g/17.5 oz	2 cups	1 gram
PurePaleo Protein	25 g/0.9 oz	1 scoop	0.1 gram

Table 4: Portion size for 30 grams of protein

Protein Source	Portion Size (Grams/Ounces)	Portion Size (Dimensions)	Saturated Fat
Egg Whites	280 g/10 oz	8 egg whites	N/A
Whole Egg	130 g/4.5 oz	6 whole eggs	18 grams
Salmon (Atlantic)	120 g/4.2 oz	12cm x 10cm x 1cm	7 grams
Salmon (Coho)	120 g/4.2 oz	12cm x 10cm x 1cm	1.2 grams
Light Tuna (in water)	120 g/4.2 oz	12cm x 10cm x 1cm	0 grams
Trout	140 g/ 4.9 oz	14cm x 10cm x 1cm	2 grams
Cod	150 g/ 5.2 oz	14cm x 10cm x 1cm	0 grams
Chicken (skinless breast)	100 g/3.5 oz	8cm x 10cm x 1cm	1 gram
Turkey (skinless breast)	100 g/3.5 oz	8cm x 10cm x 1cm	2 grams
Veal	120 g/4.5 oz	10cm x 10cm x 1cm	3.6 grams
Pork	140 g/4.9 oz	12cm x 10cm x 1cm	15 grams
Beef (lean)	90 g/3.2 oz	8cm x 10cm x 1cm	4 grams
Tofu (low fat)	360 g/12.7 oz	2 cups	2.6 grams
Whey Satisfied Protein	50 g/1.7 oz	3 scoops	0 grams
Cottage Cheese (1% fat)	240 g/8.5 oz	1 cup	3.6 grams
Greek Yogurt (0% fat)	300 g/10.5 oz	1 cup	0 grams
Regular Yogurt (2% Fat)	800 g/28 oz	3⅓ cups	2 grams
PurePaleo Protein	38 g/1.4 oz	1½ scoops	0.2 gram

FATS

Table 5: Saturated Fat Content of Different Foods

Food Source	Total Fat	Saturated Fat
1 Whole Egg	5 grams	1.6 grams
Salmon (Atlantic) 100g/3.5oz	13 grams	3 grams
Light Tuna (in water) 100g/3.5oz	0.6 grams	0 grams
Chicken (skinless breast) 100g/3.5oz	14 grams	3.8 gram
Beef (lean) 100g//3.5oz	11 grams	4.3 grams
Lamb Chop 100g/3.5oz	21 grams	9 grams
Bacon 100g/3.5oz	42 grams	14 grams
Pork Sausage 100g/3.5oz	20 grams	7 grams
10 Walnuts 15g	10 grams	1 gram
10 Cashew Nuts	9 grams	1 gram
10 Brazil Nuts	33 grams	5 grams
10 Almonds	7 grams	0.5 grams
Avocado ½ nut/75g	11 grams	1.5 grams
Whole Milk 1 cup	8 grams	5 grams
Cheddar Cheese 2tbsp/30g	8 grams	6 grams
Goat Cheese 2tbsp/30g	9 grams	6 grams
Cottage Cheese ½ cup/100g	2.5 grams	1.5 grams
Butter 1tbsp/15g	12 grams	7.3 grams
Coconut Oil 1tbsp/15g	14 grams	13 grams
Olive Oil 2tbsp/25g	25 grams	3 grams
MCT (Medium Chain Triglyceride) Oil	14 grams	14 grams
Canola Oil 2 tbsp/25g	25 grams	2 grams
Milk Chocolate 2 squares/20g	8 grams	4 grams
70% Dark Chocolate 2 squares/20g	10 grams	6 grams

CARBOHYDRATES

Table 6: Carbohydrate Content

Food	Total Carb Count	Impact Carbs	Fibre
1 bagel, 2.5 oz	38 grams	26.3 grams	1.7 grams
1 bran muffin, 2 oz	23.8 grams	19.8 grams	4 grams
1 blueberry muffin, 2 oz	27.4 grams	25.9 grams	1.5 grams
5 saltine crackers	10.7 grams	10.3 grams	0.5 grams
1 slice whole wheat bread	11.8 grams	10.7 grams	1.1 grams
1 slice white bread	14.9 grams	14.2 grams	0.7 grams
1 slice whole grain bread	11.8 grams	10.7 grams	1.1 grams
1/2 cup cooked brown rice	22.4 grams	20.6 grams	1.8 grams
1/2 cup cooked white rice	22.3 grams	21.9 grams	0.3 grams
1/2 cup cooked wild rice	17.5 grams	16 grams	1.5 grams
1/2 cup whole wheat pasta	18.6 grams	16.6 grams	2 grams
1/2 cup white pasta, cooked	20 grams	18.8 grams	1.2 grams
1/2 cup cooked oatmeal	27 grams	23 grams	4 grams
1/2 cup steel cut oats, cooked	58 grams	48 grams	10 grams
1 medium apple	25 grams	18.9 grams	4.3 grams
1 medium banana	27 grams	14.4 grams	3.1 grams
1 medium orange	16.3 grams	12.9 grams	3.4 grams
1 medium pear	25 grams	21 grams	0.5 grams
1/4 cup blueberries	5.1 grams	4.1 grams	1 gram
1/4 cup raspberries	3.6 grams	1.5 grams	2.1 grams
1/4 cup strawberries	2.7 grams	1.8 grams	1.9 grams
1/4 cup chopped dates	32.7 grams	29.4 grams	3.3 grams
1/2 cup chickpeas	22.5 grams	16.2 grams	6.2 grams
1/2 cup lentils	20 grams	12.2 grams	7.8 grams
1/2 cup corn	16 grams	14.1 grams	2 grams
1/5 cup white potato	15.4 grams	13.9 grams	1.5 grams
1/2 cup acorn squash	14.9 grams	10.4 grams	4.5 grams
1/2 cup broccoli, chopped	5.5 grams	1.1 grams	2.5 grams
1/2 cup cauliflower, chopped	5.3 grams	2.0 grams	2.1 grams

Mushrooms, 12 grams	0.6 grams	0.3 grams	0.3 grams
1 medium red pepper	7.2 grams	5 grams	2.5 grams
5 asparagus spears	3.1 grams	1 gram	1.5 grams
8 Brussels sprouts	12 grams	2.9 grams	4.4 grams

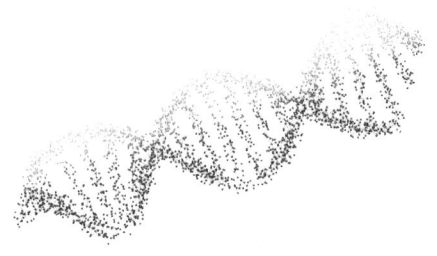

APPENDIX 2
Supplements

A Guide to the Natural Supplements Used in This Book: What They Are and Where to Get Them

The natural supplements recommended in my treatment protocols are not essential but will greatly improve your response and outcome. For many individuals, poor dietary habits will have resulted in metabolic and genetic changes that can be difficult to reverse with diet alone, which is why I incorporate supplements as part of the program for my patients. In addition, supplements can make the transition period of genetic retraining much easier and can target secondary issues such as chronic stress, which can be more difficult to control.

Supplements are available through your health-care practitioner or directly through health stores, Amazon or www.thisisgoodmedicine.com.

Note: *Before starting any supplement program, I recommend you discuss them with your health-care practitioner.*

TMC Tri-Metabolic Control™ (Douglas Laboratories)
Ingredients: Piper betle and Dolichos biflorus seed – 300 mg, acetyl-L-carnitine – 300 mg

TMC combines the clinically studied extracts of the *Piper betle* leaf and *Dolichos biflorus* seed plus acetyl-L-carnitine (ALCAR) to support three metabolic hormones—adiponectin, leptin, and ghrelin—to help control appetite, satiety and fat metabolism as part of a healthy weight management program.

Piper betle leaf and *Dolichos biflorus* seed extract have been traditionally used in Indian culture to support lipolysis. *Dolichos biflorus*, also known as horse gram, decreases oxidative stress and supports healthy lipid and glucose metabolism. *Piper betle* is an Ayurvedic herb used for blood sugar support and digestive health. The combination of the two herbs has also been clinically shown to boost adiponectin by 15% and reduce ghrelin by 17% to support healthy weight management and regulate appetite. Study results using these two herbs together at 300 milligrams three times daily combined with diet (2,000 calorie diet, so not a low-calorie diet) and exercise (moderate exercise three times a week) showed significantly reduced body weight of 9.4 pounds compared to 3.9 pounds (the group with diet and exercise only), a loss 2.4 times greater than a placebo at eight weeks, as well as an improved body mass.

Acetyl-L-carnitine (ALCAR) is a necessary component for fatty acid metabolism and energy production. It acts as a molecular shuttle in mitochondrial fatty acid oxidation, allowing fatty acids to be utilized as an energy source. It helps to improve insulin's action in muscle and regulates the production of leptin. Studies in rats (Iossa, 2002) show us the impact ALCAR has on leptin. Rats with diet-induced leptin resistance were fed 15 milligrams per litre of ALCAR in their water for one month. Diet and exercise were held constant. At the end of the month, leptin levels stabilized, and there was a significant reduction in leptin resistance. An increase in ATP production was also seen.

For more information, see www.douglaslabs.com.

Sereniten Plus (Douglas Laboratories/Pure Encapsulations)
Ingredients: Casein decapeptide (milk) (Lactium®) – 175 mg, L-Theanine (Suntheanine®) – 50 mg, vitamin D3 – 25 mcg (100 I.U.)

Sereniten Plus is a combination of casein decapeptide (Lactium®), L-Theanine and vitamin D to support the hypothalamic-pituitary-adrenal (HPA) axis and feedback, and used for stress support, cortisol regulation and weight management. Lactium® and L-Theanine have been shown to provide a calming effect and may support normal sleep that is affected by stress.

Lactium® is a bioactive decapeptide alpha-1 sequence, isolated from milk. It is effective at restoring normal HPA function and feedback. Lactium® works at three areas of the HPA axis:

- Lactium® binds specifically to the BZD site of the GABA-A receptor and does *not* bind to the PBR site of the GABA-A1 receptor responsible for the sedating effects seen with benzodiazepines.
- Lactium® increases the sensitivity of the hypothalamus to cortisol, re-establishing receptor sensitivity feedback within the HPA axis. It reduces the amount of CRH produced in response to stress.
- Lactium® decreases the amount of cortisol released by the adrenal glands during acute and chronic stress.

NOTE: Although derived from milk, Lactium® bypasses the immune system and does not induce an allergic response due to the small size of the molecule. It is therefore tolerated by those with dairy or lactose sensitivity or allergy.

L-Theanine is a unique amino acid found naturally in green tea, providing relaxation support without drowsiness. L-theanine has been shown to increase alpha-wave production in the brain, a pattern considered to be an index of relaxation.

Vitamin D has been included for additional support of immune function that may be compromised during stress. Vitamin D has many functional roles in the body, including modulation of cell growth, neuromuscular and immune function, and bone health.

For more information, see www.douglaslabs.com and www.pureencapsulations.com.

Metabolic Xtra (Pure Encapsulations)
Ingredients: Berberine HCL – 350 mg, Alpha-lipoic acid – 100 mg, resveratrol – 20 mg, chromium – 135 mcg, and vitamin C – 50 mg

Metabolic Xtra contains a combination of natural ingredients to support healthy insulin receptor function, signaling and glucose metabolism.

- The natural plant alkaloid berberine enhances the expression and function of insulin receptors to enhance glucose, lipid and triglyceride metabolism.
- Resveratrol promotes healthy AMPK and SIRT1 gene expression. These genes play important roles in fatty acid uptake and oxidation, glucose uptake by skeletal muscle and regulation of PGC1a, which increases thermogenesis.
- Zychrome™ chromium dinicocysteinate modulates cell signalling for healthy insulin function and glucose metabolism. It also provides significant support for antioxidant defense and inflammatory balance.
- Alpha-lipoic acid supports healthy receptor function and glucose metabolism.

For more information, see www.pureencapsulations.com.

Resveratrol Extra (Pure Encapsulations)
Ingredients: Japanese knotweed (Polygonum cuspidatum) *extract (standardized to 100 mg resveratrol), red wine* (Vitis vinifera) *concentrate (whole fruit) – 5 mg (standardized to contain 25% total polyphenols), grape seed extract* (Vitis vinifera) *– 50 mg (standardized to contain 92% polyphenols), ascorbyl palmitate (fat-soluble vitamin C) – 10 mg*

Resveratrol Extra combines 100 milligrams resveratrol per capsule with red wine polyphenols and grape seed extract for healthy cellular, cardiovascular and metabolic function. One capsule of Resveratrol Extra contains the same amount of resveratrol equivalent to 66 bottles of red wine.

- **Cellular health:** A recent study suggests that resveratrol may promote overall health, metabolic function and longevity. This protection may be due, at least in part, to its roles as an antioxidant and in maintaining healthy gene expression.
- **Cardiovascular support:** Resveratrol promotes cardiovascular health, helping to maintain healthy platelet function and arachidonic acid metabolism. It also helps to maintain healthy cyclooxygenase and lipoxygenase enzyme activity. Grape seed extract and red wine concentrate offer complementary polyphenols to support vascular integrity.
- **Metabolic support:** Promotes healthy AMPK and SIRT1 expression. AMPK and SIRT1 play important roles in fatty acid uptake and β-oxidation, supports glucose uptake in skeletal muscle and regulates PGC1a, which has thermogenic properties via irisin. It moderates mitochondrial output to support cellular metabolism and glucose homeostasis.

For more information, see www.pureencapsulations.com.

DopaPlus (Pure Encapsulations)
Ingredients: L-5MTHF folate as metafolin – 500 mcg, zinc – 10 mg, L-tyrosine – 1,000 mg, velvet bean (Mucuna pruriens) *extract – 200 mg (standardized to 15% L-dopa), Rhodiola extract – 100 mg (standardized to contain 3% total rosavins and minimum 1% salidrosides), grape* (Vitis vinifera) *extract seed (92% polyphenols) – 100 mg, green tea* (Camellia sinesis) *90% catechins and 70% ECGC – 100 mg, vitamin B6 in P5P form – 10 mg*

DopaPlus provides neurotransmitter precursors to help balance dopamine function in the brain for emotional wellness and to enhance daily mental function and sharpness.

- L-tyrosine and L-DOPA from *Mucuna pruriens* provide dopamine precursors.
- Vitamin B6, metafolin (L-5MTHF crosses the blood brain barrier) and zinc are synergistic cofactors that support dopamine production.
- Rhodiola with green tea polyphenols enhance dopamine binding, supports reuptake and prevents degradation.

For more information, see www.pureencapsulations.com.

Pure Lean Fiber (Pure Encapsulations)
Ingredients: Two scoops (approximately 14.4 grams) contains: 40 calories, 8 grams of carbohydrate, 6 grams of fibre, 1 gram of protein, 2 grams of sugar alcohols (from xylitol and lou han gou), 100 mg of magnesium citrate, 300 mg of naturally occurring sodium, 700 mg of PreticX™ xylooligosaacharides (a prebiotic that feeds the probiotics) and 10 grams of a proprietary fibre blend of creafibre cellulose, Sunfiber, glucomannan, prune fruit powder, flax seed fibre, apple pectin and guar gum

- Pure Lean Fiber contains a blend of prebiotics, soluble fibres from glucomannan, guar gum, apple pectin and prune powder with insoluble fibers from cellulose and flax seed to promote weight management, satiety and regularity.
- Supports healthy gut microflora with prebiotic PreticX XOS without GI side effects, while providing 6 grams of fibre and 1 gram of glucomannan.
- The gut microflora is now recognized as an important factor in overall health, with potential roles ranging from cellular and immune health to metabolic function and weight management.

For more information, see www.pureencapsulations.com.

Whey Satisfied Protein Powder (Douglas Laboratories)
Ingredients: One scoop contains: 10 grams of whey protein, 2.6 grams of Sunfiber, 1 gram of konjac gum (glucomannan), 500 mg of DNF-10

This is a unique whey protein isolate powder designed to promote satiety and weight management.

- DNF-10 is a peptide extract from *Saccharomyces cerevisiae*, clinically shown to lower NPY (neuropeptide Y) and downregulate ghrelin, thus reducing hunger and food cravings. Long-term use of DNF-10 (one month or longer) has been shown to regulate leptin to increase satiety and maximize metabolism. It also regulates insulin and glucagon-like-peptide 1 (GLP-1), helping to balance blood sugar levels and decrease cravings for carbohydrates. Studies also reveal that all weight loss using DNF-10 was adipose tissue, preserving all lean tissue mass or muscle.
- Sunfiber is a proprietary, water-soluble, non-fermentable prebiotic fibre from partially hydrolyzed guar gum that, once ingested, stretches the receptors in the stomach lining, mimicking the ingestion of food and causing an inhibition of ghrelin to reduce hunger and food-seeking behaviour. It is so powerful that is has been shown to inhibit inter-meal caloric intake or snacking by 20%.
- Glucomannan is a water-soluble fermentable fibre extract from tuber or yam. The carbohydrate type is a beta 1-4 polysaccharide chain which means this fibre passes undigested into the bowel and is then fermented by resident bacteria. It also means it is not the type of fibre that can increase blood sugar levels.
- Both fibres have also been shown to delay gastric emptying and bowel transit time, once again increasing satiety.
- All of these ingredients are mixed into 10 grams of Vanilla Spice high-grade whey protein isolate. Using this at the beginning of meals, especially lunch and dinner, decreases the desire to keep eating after meals, thus decreasing the volume of food

consumed at a meal, and helps to increase the rate of the metabolism.
- Use with other protein sources to achieve your recommended protein intake.

For more information, see www.douglaslabs.com.

PurePaleo Protein Powder (Designs for Health)
Ingredients: One scoop provides 21 grams of protein plus vitamins A and D

PurePaleo is a dairy-free protein powder made from proprietary hydrolyzed beef (HydroBEEF), a concentrated bone broth protein isolate. The protein peptides are hydrolyzed or broken down in such a way as to maximize absorption and assimilation. It contains a significant amount of collagen to help support joints and skin, along with extra fat-soluble vitamins A and D. It is ideal for people who are sensitive to dairy, rice or soy.

For more information, see www.designsforhealth.ca.

Arthroben (Designs for Health)
Ingredients: Collagen peptides (Fortigel and Verisol), bioflavonoids (baicalin and catcechin)

Arthroben is a highly absorbable powder comprised of the hydrolyzed collagen peptides Fortigel and Verisol plus bioflavonoids baicalin from *Scuttelaria baicalenis* and catcechin from *Acacia catechu*. These extracts are designed to support and strengthen connective tissue and joints. Arthroben provides hydrolyzed collagen peptides that act as building blocks to repair damaged cartilage, ligaments and skin, along with natural bioflavonoids that inhibit COX-1, COX-2 and 5-LOX inflammatory pathways.

For more information, see www.designsforhealth.ca.

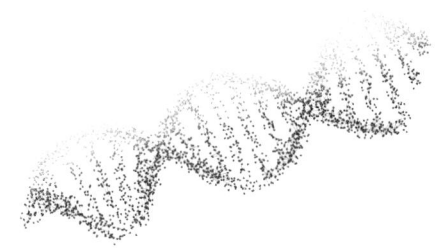

APPENDIX 3
Resources

https://www.GeneRx.ca
GeneRx.ca is an online integrated SNP interpretation program that allows your health-care practitioner or personal trainer to upload 23andMe data and obtain a personalized health analysis and treatment protocol.
www.generx.ca

pkrhealth.ca
Dr. Penny Kendall-Reed Naturopathic Doctor website.

Commercial SNP genotyping websites:
https://www.23andMe.com
https://www.ancestry.ca
https://www.livingdna.com
https://www.myheritage.com
https://www.orig3n.com
https://www.homedna.com
https://www.crigenetics.com
https://www.fitnessgenes.com

National Human Genome Research Institute
Genome-Wide Association Studies Fact Sheet
https://www.genome.gov/about-genomics/fact-sheets/Genome-Wide-Association-Studies-Fact-Sheet

SNPedia is an online SNP database:
www.SNPedia.com

dbSNP is an online National Institutes of Health SNP database:
https://www.ncbi.nlm.nih.gov/snp/

Websites for Product Purchase by Health-Care Practitioners:
www.pureencapsulations.com
www.douglaslabs.com
www.designsforhealth.com

Websites for Product Purchase by Everyone:
www.thisisgoodmedicine.com
www.amazon.ca
Local health food shops

For personalized recipes and meal plans catered to your specific genetics, see:
www.feedyourgenes.com

Books
The New Naturopathic Diet (Winding Star Press, 2002, ISBN: 1 55082 302 7)
The No Crave Diet (Virgin Books, 2008, ISBN: 978 0 7535 1313 2)
The Complete Doctor's Stress Solution (Robert Rose Inc. 2004, ISBN 0 7788 0096 2)
Healing Arthritis (Quarry Press Inc. 2002, ISBN 1 55082 312 4)
The Complete Doctor's Healthy Back Bible (Robert Rose Inc. 2004, ISBN 0 7788 0091 1)

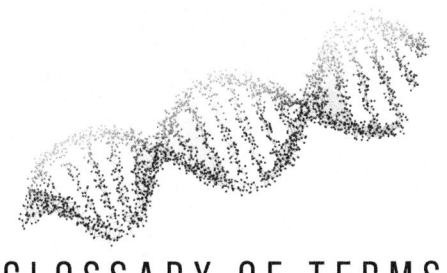

GLOSSARY OF TERMS

α-MSH: Alpha-melanocyte stimulating hormone. One of the major satiety or anti-hunger messengers in the brain.

Adipokine: Any of a number of messenger hormones produced by fat cells, for example, leptin.

Adiponectin: A hormone produced by fat cells that regulates insulin sensitivity and the metabolism and storage of fats, and reduces inflammation.

Adipose tissue: The fat storage tissue in your body.

Adrenal glands: Glands that sit above each kidney and produce hormone messengers including cortisol.

AGRP (agouti-related peptide): One of the hunger messengers in the brain.

Allele: A variant form of a gene. As humans have two copies of each gene, we have two alleles, one inherited from each parent.

Amino acids: The individual molecules that are assembled into long chains to form proteins.

Amygdala: An area of the brain involved with emotional response and reaction to stress.

Autonomic nervous system: The part of the nervous system that is not under conscious or voluntary control. It is responsible for functions such as blood pressure, heart rate and sweating, among others.

Basal metabolic rate: The rate at which the body expends energy for basic activities of living, including organ function and breathing.

Base Pair: The "rungs" of the DNA double-helix molecule comprise bonded pairs of the nucleic acids, guanine, cytosine, adenine and thymine.

Blood sugar: The concentration of sugar (glucose) molecules in your bloodstream.

BMI: See Body Mass Index

Body Mass Index (BMI): A basic measure of obesity determined by dividing your body weight in kilograms by the square of your height in metres. Although measured in units of kg/m^2 BMI is often represented simply as a number without units.

For example, if your weight is 65 kilograms and your height is 1.67 metres, then your BMI = $65/1.67^2$ = 23.

As a measure of health:
BMI < 18.5   Underweight
BMI = 18.5 to 24.9   Normal weight
BMI = 25 to 29.9   Overweight
BMI > 30   Obese

Calorie: A measure of the amount of energy available from food.

Carbohydrate: A food type containing chains of sugar molecules.

CART: Cocaine and amphetamine related transcript. A protein messenger molecule in the brain associated with hunger and reward.

Central nervous system: The main part of the nervous system that includes the spinal cord and brain.

Central obesity: Accumulation of fat around the abdominal or trunk area.

Cholecystokinin (CCK): An important satiety messenger released in the gut when you eat.

Chromosome: The structure within cells into which DNA is organized.

Coding strand: The DNA strand that holds the code for the protein manufactured by each gene. It also called the mRNA-like strand, the sense strand or the positive (+) strand. (See DNA Strand Terminology on page 29).

Codon: A sequence of three nucleotides, which together form a unit of genetic code for an amino acid in a DNA or RNA molecule.

Complex carbohydrates: Carbohydrate sources that are not easily broken down and absorbed as simple sugars, which includes vegetables, salads and legumes (see **Low Glycemic**).

Corticotrophin-releasing hormone (CRH): A stress messenger in the brain that causes an increase in cortisol in the bloodstream.

Cortisol: The body's major stress hormone produced by the adrenal glands.

DNA: Deoxyribonucleic acid is the molecule within cells that makes up chromosomes. It carries your individual genetic information.

DNA orientation: Allele coding can vary between platforms for the same SNP. Most of the time this relates to which DNA strand is referenced; the coding (+) strand or the template (-) strand. As nucleotides are in pairs (A-T and G-C), what may be an A-allele on one strand is automatically a T-allele on the other. This variability is termed "strand orientation."

DNA strand: The DNA molecule has two strands, like the sides of a ladder, connected by nucleic acid base-pair "rungs". (See DNA Strand Terminology on page 29).

Dominant: A term applied to an allele if it is expressed in a person who has only one copy of that allele. It overpowers a recessive allele (see also **Recessive**).

Dopamine: An important chemical messenger in the brain.

Downregulation: Lowered activity of a hormone or chemical messenger resulting from a decrease in the number of receptors for that hormone or chemical. Turns the message "off".

DRD2: D2 dopamine receptor in the brain.

Dyslipidemia: An excessive amount of lipids including cholesterol and triglycerides in the blood. Also termed hyperlipidemia. Associated with numerous adverse health effects.

Endocrine glands: Organs of the body containing specialized cells that secrete hormones, for example, the pancreas, which secretes insulin.

Epigenetics: The field of study that looks at how external factors such as diet, stress and the environment can affect the expression of genes.

Exon: A segment of DNA within a gene that contains the actual coding information for a protein (see also **Intron**).

Expression: The degree to which a gene produces the protein for which it codes.

Fight-or-flight response: The series of reactions or events designed to help the body handle acute stress.

GABA (gaba-aminobutyric acid): A neurotransmitter involved in the reward system.

Gene: A specific section of DNA that is responsible for coding for a protein.

Genome: The entire human DNA set including all genes.

Genotype: The genetic coding for a particular gene. It can refer to one or all genes.

Genotyping: A DNA analysis technique that searches for specific variants within an individual's DNA.

GI tract: The gastro-intestinal tract or digestive system extending from the mouth to the anus.

GWAS (genome-wide association study): Genome-wide association studies are a research tool used to identify genes that are involved in the development or progression of human disease.

Haplotype: Half of your entire DNA set and inherited from one parent. It is equivalent to half your **Genotype**. Can also refer to a cluster of inheritable **single nucleotide polymorphisms (SNPs)**.

HDL: High-density lipoprotein. Also called "good cholesterol."

Heterozygote: An individual that has two different alleles for a particular gene.

Heterozygous: The situation in which the two alleles for a particular gene are different.

High glycemic: Term used for carbohydrate foods that are easily broken down and rapidly absorbed into the bloodstream, which includes simple forms of sugar such as glucose, lactose and fructose and starchy foods such as bread, potatoes, fruit and sweets (see **Simple carbohydrates**).

HIIT: High-intensity interval training. A form of exercise training that alternates vigorous bouts of activity such as sprinting with lower intensity recovery periods.

Homeostasis: The tendency toward a relatively stable equilibrium between interdependent elements, especially as maintained by physiological processes.

Homozygote: An individual in whom the two alleles of a particular gene are the same.

Homozygous: The situation in which the two alleles for a particular gene are the same.

HPA axis: An acronym for the hypothalamic-pituitary-adrenal axis or stress pathway.

Hunger centre: The region of the brain that when active makes you feel hungry.

Hyperglycemia: A concentration of glucose molecules in your blood that is higher than normal.

Hypoglycemia: A low concentration of sugar molecules in your bloodstream.

Hyperinsulinemia: Persistently high insulin levels in the blood.

Hypothalamus: A small but important area of the brain responsible for controlling numerous primitive mechanisms including hunger, stress and satiety.

Insulin: A hormone produced by the pancreas that lowers blood sugar and stores fat.

Insulin resistance: A condition in which the body is insensitive and even resistant to the effects of insulin. In most cases, the body responds by producing even more insulin, leading to **Hyperinsulinemia**.

Intron: A segment of DNA within a gene that contains non-coding information for a protein. This type of information may relate to guiding expression or transcription of the gene, for example, or to be redundant information (see also **Exon**).

Ketosis: A dietary state usually associated with starvation in which the body primarily uses fatty acids and ketone bodies rather than glucose as fuel.

Legume: Foods such as beans, peas, chickpeas and lentils. Considered **Complex carbohydrates** with a **Low glycemic** index. They contain a high carbohydrate-to-protein ratio.

LDL: Low-density lipoprotein. Also called "bad cholesterol."

Leptin: A hormone produced by fat cells that decreases appetite and increases energy expenditure.

Leptin resistance: Resistance of the body to the effects of leptin.

Lipid: Fat or fatty substances including fatty acids, oils, waxes and steroids hormones.

Lipogenesis: The formation of fat and the transformation of non-fat materials into body fat.

Low glycemic: Term used for carbohydrates that are not broken down easily into sugars. Thus, sugar release into the bloodstream is slower. Low-glycemic foods include vegetables, salads and legumes (see **Complex carbohydrates**).

Major allele: The most common allele within a population, which is usually (but not always) the normal allele.

MC4R: Melanocortin-4 receptor.

Metabolic syndrome: A disease complex characterized by central obesity, high blood pressure, insulin resistance, type 2 diabetes, increased cholesterol and increased risk of heart disease and stroke.

Metabolism: The overall term for the on-going chemical processes in the body that burn food and produce energy.

Methylation: An inheritable chemical modification of DNA that affects gene expression.

Minor allele: The less common allele within a population, which is usually (but not always) the risk or variant allele.

Monogenic: A trait that is controlled by one gene (see **Polygenic**).

mRNA: Messenger RNA

Mutation: A permanent and heritable alteration in the DNA sequence that makes up a gene causing it to be different from the normal or baseline sequence.

Neuropeptide-Y (NPY): The hunger messenger in the brain that increases hunger, food cravings and fat storage.

Neurotransmitter: A chemical messenger within the brain or nervous system.

Normal allele: Typically the original or baseline allele and normally not associated with increased risk. It is also called: ancestral allele, standard allele, wild allele, reference allele, **Major allele**.

Nucleic Acid: See **Nucleotide base**.

Nucleotide base: One of the basic structural building blocks of DNA or RNA. They are adenine, guanine, cytosine and thymine (uracil in RNA).

Nutrigenomics: The study of interactions between diet/nutrition and gene expression.

Nutritional supplementation: The use of vitamins, minerals and herbs for preventive and therapeutic purposes.

Obesity: An excessive accumulation of body fat in subcutaneous and visceral tissues. It is generally considered to occur when a person has a BMI (**Body Mass Index**) of 30 and above. It is a complex condition associated with numerous health issues.

Odds Ratio: The Odds Ratio is a statistical value that quantifies whether one event is likely to lead to another, that is, how closely two events are associated. For example, using the lung cancer figures: if 17% or 17 out of 100 individuals exposed to smoking develop lung cancer then the odds of developing the disease in smokers is 17 divided by 83 (number that smoked but didn't get cancer), which equals 0.205. Only 1 in 100 non-smokers develop cancer so the odds in this group is 0.01. The Odds Ratio is the first figure divided by the second, 0.205/0.01, which equals 20.5. If this figure were 1, then it could be said that smoking does not affect lung cancer. If the number is greater than 1, then smoking leads to a higher risk of cancer. The greater this number is, the higher the risk. Thus, 20 is very high.

Orexins: A group of appetite-stimulating chemical messengers.

Orientation: See **DNA Orientation**.

Phenotype: The human effect of our gene coding (**Genotype**). This can be anything from appearance (such as eye colour) to functions such as metabolism (increased tendency to store fat) and disease risk (diabetes, for example).

Polygenic: A trait that is influenced by a number of genes (see **Monogenic**).

POMC: Propriomelanocortin. A protein messenger molecule in the brain associated with hunger and satiety.

Protein: A food type containing chains of amino acids that is used primarily to rebuild the body and produce many important molecules such as hormones and enzymes.

Receptors: Membrane-bound molecules with specific sites for other molecules such as hormones and neurotransmitters to bind into.

Recessive: A term applied to an allele if it is only expressed in a person who has two copies of that allele. It is overpowered by a dominant allele (see also **Dominant**).

Relative Risk (also called Risk Ratio): Relative Risk is a value that defines the ratio of the likelihood of an event occurring in a test or exposed group versus the likelihood of the event occurring in a control or non-exposed group. For example, if the risk of developing lung cancer in smokers (exposed group) is 17% and the risk in non-smokers (non-exposed or control group) is 1%, then the Relative Risk of developing lung cancer in smokers is 17 divided by 1, which equals 17. Smokers are 17 times more likely to develop lung cancer.

RNA: Ribonucleic acid. A messenger molecule created from DNA through **Transcription**. It carries instructions to control the synthesis of a protein.

rs number: A reference number used to refer to a specific SNP (**Single Nucleotide Polymorphism**). It stands for Reference SNP cluster ID.

Satiety: The sensation of feeling "full" and no longer hungry.

Satiety centre: The region of the brain that when active makes you feel full.

Sequencing: The process to determine the exact sequence of a DNA strand.

Serotonin: A chemical messenger important in the control of mood and craving.

Simple carbohydrate: A simple form of sugar such as glucose, lactose and fructose, which is rapidly absorbed into the bloodstream. Simple carbohydrates include foods such as bread, potatoes, fruit and sweets.

SNP (single nucleotide polymorphism): A SNP (pronounced "snip") is a difference in a single nucleotide of one base pair in a DNA sequence. For example, at a specific locus in a gene the population might show two different sequences:

TGG**C**AG or TGG**T**AG

In this case, there would be a SNP at position 4. As opposed to mutations, SNPs are extremely common.

SNPedia: An online, publically available resource that provides a database of known single nucleotide polymorphisms (SNPs).

Template strand: The DNA strand that is used as a template to make mRNA. Also called the anti-sense strand or negative (-) strand. (See DNA Strand Terminology on page 29).

Trait: A particular characteristic of an individual that is the result of certain genetic coding, for example, eye colour.

Transcription: The process by which the information in a strand of DNA is copied into a new molecule of messenger RNA (mRNA).

Translation: The process by which a molecule of messenger RNA (mRNA) is used to construct a protein molecule.

Upregulation: Heightened activity of a hormone or chemical messenger resulting from an increase in the number of receptors for that hormone or chemical. Turns the message "on."

Variant allele: Typically, the abnormal or risk allele for a SNP. It is also called: risk allele, derived allele, mutant allele, atypical allele, **Minor allele**.

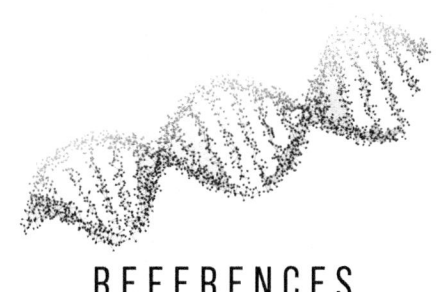

REFERENCES

Background for Chapters 1 to 4 and Conclusion

Ashan M. et al. 2017. "The relative contribution of DNA methylation and genetic variants on protein biomarkers for human diseases." *PLOS Genetics*.doi.org/10.1371/journal.pgen.1007005.

Bjornsson H. et al. 2015. "Histone deacetylase inhibition rescues structural and functional brain deficits in a mouse model of Kabuki syndrome." *Sci. Transl. Med.* 6(256): 256.

Breton C.V. et al. 2014. "Air pollution and epigenetics: Recent findings." *Curr. Envir. Health Rpt.* 1: 35.

Cao-Lei L. et al. 2014. "DNA methylation signatures triggered by prenatal maternal stress exposure to a natural disaster: Project Ice Storm." *PLOS One* 19(9): e107653.

Chamberlain A. et al. 2009. "Ala54Thr polymorphism of the fatty acid binding protein 2 gene and saturated fat intake in relation to lipid levels and insulin resistance: The Coronary Artery Risk Development in Young Adults (CARDIA) study." *Metabolism* 58(9): 1222–1228.

Christiaans I. et al. 2011. "Germline SMARCB1 mutation and somatic NF2 mutations in familial multiple meningiomas." *J. Med. Genet.* 48: 93–97.

Clair D. et al. 2005. "Rates of adult schizophrenia following prenatal exposure to the Chinese famine of 1959–1961." *JAMA* 294(5): 557–562.

De Oliveira C. et al. 2011. "High-fat diet and glucocorticoid treatment cause hyperglycemia associated with adiponectin receptor alteration." *Lipids in Health and Disease* 10: 11.

De Prins S. et al. 2013. "Influence of ambient air pollution on global DNA methylation in healthy adults: A seasonal follow-up." *Environment International* 59: 418–424.

Dias B. et al. 2014. "Parental olfactory experience influences behavior and neural structure in subsequent generations." *Nature Neuroscience* 17: 89–96.

Dinga R. et al. 2016. "H3K9 acetylation change patterns in rats after exposure to traffic-related air pollution." *Environmental Toxicology and Pharmacology* 42: 170–175.

Duse J.A. et al. 2008. "Genomic counter-stress changes induced by the relaxation response." *PLOS One* Jul 2.3(7): e2576.

Glad C. et al. 2017. "Reduced DNA methylation and psychopathology following endogenous hyper cortisolism – A genome-wide study." *Scientific Reports* 7: article number 44445.

Gorlove O. et al. 2012. "Derived SNP alleles are used more frequently than ancestral alleles as risk-associated variants in common human diseases." *J. Bioinform. Comput. Biol.* 10(2): 1241008.

Heijmans B. et al. 2008. "Persistent epigenetic differences associated with prenatal exposure to famine in humans." *Proc. Natl. Acad. Sci.* 105(44): 17046–17049.

Hershey A. et al. 1952. "Independent functions of viral protein and nucleic acid in growth of bacteriophage." *J. Gen. Physiol.* 36(1): 39–56.

Horvath S. 2013. "DNA methylation age of human tissues and cell types." *Genome Biol.* 14(10): R115.

Jones M. et al. 2013. "DNA methylation, genotype and gene expression: Who is driving and who is along for the ride?" *Genome Biol.* 14(7): 126.

Jones S. et al. 2015. "Personalized genomic analyses for cancer mutation discovery and interpretation." *Sci. Transl. Med.* 7(283): 283ra53.

Karki R. et al. 2015. "Standards and guidelines for the interpretation of sequence variants: A joint consensus recommendation of the American College of Medical Genetics and Genomics and the Association for Molecular Pathology." *Genet. Med.* 17: 405–423.

Kendall-Reed P. and Reed S. 2002. *The New Naturopathic Diet*. Winding Star Press ISBN: 1–55082–302–7.

Kendall-Reed P. and Reed S. 2008. *The No Crave Die*t. Virgin Books ISBN: 978–0–7535–1313–2.

Kendall-Reed P. and Reed S. 2004. *The Complete Doctor's Stress Solution*. Robert Rose Inc. ISBN: 0–7788–0096–2.

Klein R.J. et al. 2005. "Complement factor H polymorphism in age-related macular degeneration." *Science* 308(5720): 385-389.

Leone O. et al. 2006. "A human derived SSADH coding variant is replacing the ancestral allele shared with primates." *Ann. Hum. Biol.* 33(5-6): 593–603.

Lester B. et al. 2018. "Epigenetic programming by maternal behavior in the human infant." *Pediatrics* 142(4): e20171890.

Liu X.S. et al. 2016. "Editing DNA methylation in the mammalian genome." *Cell* 167: 233–247.

Malki K. et al. 2016. "Epigenetic differences in monozygotic twins discordant for major depressive disorder." *Transl. Psychiatry* 6(6): e839.

Meer M. et al. 2018. "A whole lifespan mouse multi-tissue DNA methylation clock." *Elife* 7: e40675.

Moore L. et al. 2013. "DNA Methylation and Its Basic Function." *Neuropsychopharm.* 38(1): 23–38.

Naisbitt J. 1982. *Megatrends: ten new directions transforming our lives.* New York Warner Books ISBN: 0446512516.

National Human Genome Research Institute. Bethesda, MD USA 2015 https://www.genome.gov/about-genomics/fact-sheets/Genome-Wide-Association-Studies-Fact-Sheet.

Osaki K and Tanaka T. 2006. "Genome-wide association study to identify single nucleotide polymorphisms conferring risk of myocardial infarction." *Methods Mol. Med.* 128: 173-180.

Painter R.C. et al. 2005. "Prenatal exposure to the Dutch famine and disease in later life: An overview." *Reproductive Toxicology* 20: 345–352.

Park S. et al. 2016. "Interactions with the MC4R rs17782313 variant, mental stress and energy intake and the risk of obesity in Genome Epidemiology Study." *Nutrition & Metabolism* 13: 38.

Phillips C.M. et al. 2012. "March 2012 Dietary saturated fat, gender and genetic variation at the TCF7L2 locus predict the development of metabolic syndrome." *J. Nutr. Biochem.* 23(3): 239–244.

Rands C. et al. 2014. "8.2% of the human genome Is constrained: Variation in rates of turnover across functional element classes in the human lineage." *PLOS Genetics* 10(7): e1004525.

Rodgers A. et al. 2013. "Paternal stress exposure alters sperm microRNA content and reprograms offspring HPA stress axis regulation." *J. Neurosci.* 33(21): 9003–9012.

Rojas D. et al. 2015. "Prenatal arsenic exposure and the epigenome: Identifying sites of 5-methylcytosine alterations that predict functional changes in gene expression in newborn cord blood and subsequent birth outcomes." *Toxicological Sciences* 143(1): 97–106.

Roy S. et al. 2005. "Wound site neutrophil transcription in response to psychological stress in young men." *Gene Expression* 12(4–6): 273–287.

Ryan J. et al. 2007. "The relationship between non-protein-coding DNA and eukaryotic complexity." *Bioessays* 29(3): 288–299.

Saeden N. et al. 2017. "Lower placental Leptin promoter methylation in association with fine particulate matter air pollution during pregnancy and placental nitrosative stress at birth in the ENVIRONAGE cohort." *Environmental Health Perspectives* 125(2): 262–268.

Schulz L. and Chaudhari L. 2015. "High risk populations: The Pima Indians of Arizona and Mexico." *Curr. Obes. Rep.* 4(1): 92–98.

Shimazu T. et al. 2013. "Suppression of oxidative stress by beta-hydroxybutyrate, an endogenous histone deacetylase inhibitor." *Science* 11,339(6116): 211–214.

Sofer T. et al. 2013. "Exposure to airborne particulate matter is associated with methylation pattern in the asthma pathway." *Epigenomics* 5: 147–154.

Swartz J.R. et al. 2017. "An epigenetic mechanism links socioeconomic status to changes in depression-related brain function in high-risk adolescents." *Mol. Psychiatry* 22(2): 209–214.

Watson J. and Crick F. 1953. "Molecular structure of nucleic acids: A structure for deoxyribose nucleic acid." *Nature* 171: 737–738.

Welcome Trust Case Control Consortium, 2007. "Genome-wide association study of 14,000 cases of seven common disease and 3,000 shared controls." *Nature* 447(7145): 661–678.

Vinkers C.H. et al. 2015. "Traumatic stress and human DNA methylation: A critical review." *Epigenomics* 7(4): 593–608.

Yehuda R. et al. 2016. "Holocaust exposure induced intergenerational effects on FKBP5 methylation." *Biol. Psych.* 80(5): 372–380.

Background for FTO

Ahmad T. et al. 2011. "Lifestyle interaction with fat mass and obesity-associated (*FTO*) genotype and risk of obesity in apparently healthy U.S. women." *Diabetes Care* 34(3): 675–680.

Andreasen C.H. et al. 2008. "Low physical activity accentuates the effect of the FTO rs9939609 polymorphism on body fat accumulation." *Diabetes* 57: 95–101.

Austin J. et al. 2009. "Hormonal regulators of appetite." *Int. J Pediatr. Endocrinol*. 2009: 141753.

Burger K.S. et al. 2014. "A functional neuroimaging review of obesity, appetitive hormones and ingestive behaviour." *Physiol. Behav.* 136: 121–127.

Claussnitzer M. et al. 2015. "FTO obesity variant circuitry and adipocyte browning in humans." *N. Engl. J. Med.* 373: 895–907.

Corella D. et al. 2011. "A high intake of saturated fatty acids strengthens the association between the fat mass and obesity-associated gene and BMI". *J. Nutr.* 141(12): 2219–2225.

Drolet R. et al. 2009. "Fat depot-specific impact of visceral obesity on adipocyte adiponectin release in women." 17(3): 424–430.

Fang H. et al. 2010. "Variant rs9939609 in the FTO gene is associated with body mass index among Chinese children." *BCM Medical Genetics* 11: 136.

Fawcett K. et al. 2010 "The genetics of obesity: Obesity leads the way." *Trends Genet.* 26(6): 266-274.

Frayling T. et al. 2007. "A common variant in FTO gene is associated with body mass index and predisposes to childhood and adult obesity." *Science* 316(5826): 889-894.

Iossa S. et al. 2002. "Acetyl-L-Carntine supplementation differently influences nutrient partitioning, serum Leptin concentration and skeletal muscle mitochondrial respiration in young and old rats." *J. Nutr.* 132(4): 636-642

Jia G. et al. "N6-Methyladenosine in nuclear RNA is a major of obesity-associated in FTO." *Nat. Chem. Biol.* 7(12): 885–887.

Karra E. et al. 2013. "A link between FTO, ghrelin, and impaired brain food-cue responsivity." *J. Clin. Invest.* 123(8): 3539–3551.

Labayen I. et al. 2011. "Association between the FTO rs9939609 polymorphism and Leptin in European adolescents: A possible link with energy balance control. The HELENA study." *Int. J. Obesity (Lond.)* 35(1): 66–71.

Magno F. et al. 2018. "Influence of *FTO* rs9939609 polymorphism on appetite, ghrelin, Leptin, IL6, TNFα levels, and food intake of women with morbid obesity." *Diabetes Metab. Syndr. Obes.* 11: 199–207.

Moghanloo M. et al. 2018. "Polymorphism rs9939609 of fat mass and obesity-associated gene correlation with leptin level of obese women suffered from type 2 diabetes." *Curr. Diabetes Rev.* 14(6): 559–564.

Naleid A.M. et al. 2005. "Ghrelin induces feeding in the mesolimbic reward pathway between the ventral tegmental area and the nucleus accumbens." *Peptides* 26(11): 2274–2279.

Nigro E. et al. 2014. "New insight into adiponectin role in obesity and obesity-related diseases." *Biomed. Res. Int.* Epub. 658913.

Perello M. et al. 2012. "Functional implications of limited Leptin receptor and ghrelin receptor coexpression in the brain." *J. Comp. Neurol.* 520(2): 281–294.

Qi L. et al. 2008. "Fat mass-and obesity-associated (FTO) gene variant is associated with obesity: Longitudinal analyses in two cohort studies and functional test." *Diabetes* 57(11): 3145–3151.

Ronkainen J. et al. 2015. "Fat mass and obesity-associated gene FTO affects the dietary response in mouse white adipose tissue." *Scientific Reports* 5: 9233.

Sandholt C.H. et al. 2012. "Beyond the fourth wave of genome-wide obesity association studies." *Nutr. Diabetes* 2: 37.

Schwartz M.W. et al. 2000. "Central nervous system control of food intake." *Nature* 404(6778): 661–671.

Smemo S. et al. 2014. "Obesity-associated variants within FTO from long-range functional connections with IRX3." *Nature* 507(7492): 371–375.

Stern J. et al. 2016. "Adiponectin, leptin, and fatty acids in the maintenance of metabolic homeostasis through adipose tissue crosstalk." *Cell Metabolism* 23(5): 770–784.

Veldhuis J.D. et al. 2010. "Integrating GHS into the ghrelin system." *Int. J. Pept.* 2010: 879503.

Yang Y. et al. 2016. "*FTO* genotype and type 2 diabetes mellitus: Spatial analysis and meta-analysis of 62 case-control studies from different regions." *Genes (Basel)* 8(2): 70.

Background for ADIPOQ

Arnav K. et al. 2016. "Evolving role of adiponectin in cancer-controversies and update." *Cancer Biol. Med.* 13(1): 101–119.

Cawthorn W.P. et al. 2014. "Bone marrow adipose tissue is an endocrine organ that contributes to increased circulating adiponectin during caloric restriction." *Cell Metab.* 20(2): 368–375.

Christina L. et al. 2011. "Associations of SNPs in ADIPOQ and subclinical cardiovascular disease in the Multi-Ethnic Study of Atherosclerosis (MESA)." *Obesity* (Silver Spring) 19(4): 840–847.

Cui M. et al. 2016. "Association of ADIPOQ single nucleotide polymorphisms with the risk of intracranial atherosclerosis." *Int. J. Neurosci.* 127(5): 1–19.

De Oliveira C. et al. 2011. "High-fat diet and glucocorticoid treatment cause hyperglycemia associated with adiponectin receptor alterations." *Lipids Health Dis.* 10: 11.

Fallo F. et al. 2004. "Effect of glucocorticoids on adiponectin: A study in healthy subjects and in Cushing's syndrome." *Eur. J Endocrinol.* 150(3): 339–344.

Goldstein B. et al. 2009. "Protective vascular and myocardial effects of adiponectin." *Nature Clin. Prac. Cardiovasc. Med.* 6: 27–35 (https://www.nature.com/articles/ncpcardio1398).

Goyenechea E. et al. 2009. "The - 11391 G/A polymorphism of the adiponectin gene promoter Is associated with metabolic syndrome traits and the outcome of an energy-restricted diet in obese subjects." *Horm. Metab. Res.* 41: 55–61.

Heid I.M. et al. 2010. "Clear detection of ADIPOQ locus as the major gene for plasma adiponectin: Results of genome-wide association analyses including 4659 European individuals." *Atherosclerosis* 208(2): 412–420.

Ishikawa M. et al. 2005. "Plasma adiponectin and gastric cancer." *Clin. Cancer Res.* 11: 466–472.

Lee S. and Kwak H. 2014. "Role of adiponectin in metabolic and cardiovascular disease." *J. Exerc. Rehabil.* 10(2): 54–59.

Ouchi N. et al. 1999. "Novel modulator for endothelial adhesion molecules: Adipocyte-derived plasma protein adiponectin." *Circulation* 100: 2473–2476.

Ukkola O. et al. 2002. "Adiponectin: A link between excess adiposity and associated comorbidities?" *J. Mol.* 80(11): 696–702.

Yamauchi T. et al. 2001. "The fat-derived hormone adiponectin reverses insulin resistance associated with both lipoatrophy and obesity." *Nat. Med.* 7(8): 941–946.

Background for MC4R

Blum K. et al. 2014. "Dopamine and glucose, obesity and reward deficiency syndrome." *Front Psychol.* 25: 919.

Chambers J.C. et al. 2008. "Common genetic variation near MC4R is associated with waist circumference and insulin resistance." *Nat. Genet.* 40(6): 716–718.

Davis C. et al. 2012. "Binge eating disorder and the dopamine D2 receptor: Genotypes and sub-phenotypes." *Prog. Neuopsychopharmacol. Biol. Psychiatry* 38(2): 328–335.

Davis J. et al. 2011. "Central melancortins modulate mesocorticolimbic activity and food seeking behaviour in the rat." *Physiol. Behav.* 102(5): 491–495.

Farooqi I.S. et al. 2003. "Clinical spectrum of obesity and mutations in the melanocortin 4 receptor gene." *N. Engl. J Med.* 348(12): 1085.

Greenfield J. et al. 2009. "Modulation of blood pressure by central melanocortinergic pathways." *N. Engl. J. Med. 360(1): 44–52.*

Hinney A. et al. 2013, "Melanocortin-4 Receptor in homeostasis and obesity pathogenesis." *Prog. Mol. Biol. Transl. Sci.* 114: 147–191.

Leońska-Duniec A. et al. 2017. "Impact of the polymorphism near MC4R (rs17782313) on obesity and metabolic-related traits in women participating in an aerobic training program." *J. Hum. Kinet.* 58: 111–119.

Lim B.K. et al. 2012. "Anhedonia requires MC4R-mediated synaptic adaptations in nucleus accumbens." *Nature* 487: 183–189.

Marcadenti A. et al. 2013. "Effects of FTO rs9939906 and MC4R rs17782313 on obesity, type 2 diabetes mellitus and blood pressure in patients with hypertension." *Cardiovasc. Diabet.* 12: 103.

Marks D.L. et al. 2004. "Ala67Thr polymorphism in the agouti-related peptide gene is associated with inherited leanness in humans." *Am. J. Med. Genet.* 126: 267–271.

Meyre D. et al. 2009. "Genome-wide association study for early-onset and morbid adult obesity identifies three new risk loci in European populations." *Net. Genet.* 41(2): 157–159.

Park S. et al. 2016. "Interactions with the MC4R rs17782313 variant, mental stress and energy intake and the risk of obesity in Genome Epidemiology Study." *Nutrit. Metab.* 13: 38.

Qui L. et al. 2008. "The common obesity variant near MC4R gene is associated with higher intakes of total energy and dietary fat, weight change and diabetes risk in women." *Hum. Mol. Genet.* 17(22): 3502–3508.

Ren X. et al. 2010. "Nutrient selection in the absence of taste receptor signalling." *J. Neurosci.* 30(23): 8012–8023.

Tallam L.S. et al. 2005. "Melanocortin-4 receptor deficient mice are not hypertensive or salt sensitive despite obesity, hyperinsulinaemia and hyperleptinaemia." *Hypertension* 46(2): 326–332.

Tschritter O. et al. 2011. "An obesity risk SNP (rs17782313) near the MC4R gene is associated with cerebrocortical insulin resistance in humans." *J. Obes.* 2011: 283153.

Willer C.J. et al. 2009. "Six new loci associated with body mass index highlight a neuronal influence on body weight regulation." *Nat. Genet.* 41(1): 25–34.

Ya-Xiong T. 2010. "The Melanocortin-4 receptor: Physiology, pharmacology, and pathophysiology." *Endocr. Rev.* 31(4): 506–543.

Yilmaz Z. et al. 2015. "Association between MC4R rs17782313 polymorphism and overeating behaviours." *International Journal of Obesity* 39(1): 114–120.

Yoon Y.R. et al. 2015. "Melancortin 4 receptor and dopamine D2 receptor expression in brain areas involved in food intake." *Endocrinol. Metab.* (Seoul). 30(4): 576–583.

Background for PPARG

Deeb S. et al. 1998. "A Pro12Ala substitution in PPARgamma2 associated with decreased receptor activity, lower body mass index and improved insulin sensitivity." *Nat Genet.* 20(3): 284–287.

Julie A. et al. 2001. "The Peroxisome Poliferator–Activated receptor-γ2 Pro12Ala variant association with type 2 diabetes and trait differences." *Diabetes* 50(4): 886–890.

Kawai M. et al. 2010. "PPARγ: A circadian transcription factor in adipogenesis and osteogenesis." *Nat. Rev. Endocrinol.* 6(11): 629–636.

Kilpeläinen T. et al. 2008. "SNPs in PPARG associate with type 2 diabetes and interact with physical activity." *Med. Sci. Sports Exerc.* 40(1): 25–33.

Lee M. et al. 2018. "New insight of high-intensity interval training on physiological adaptation with brain functions." <u>*J. Exerc. Nutrition Biochem*</u>. 22(3): 1–5.

López-Alarcón M. et al. 2012. "PPARγ2 Pro12Ala polymorphism is associated with improved lipoprotein lipase functioning in adipose tissue of insulin resistant obese women." *Gene* 511(2): 404–410.

Luan J. et al. 2001. "Evidence for gene-nutrient interaction at the PPARgamma locus." *Diabetes* 50(3): 686–689.

Mansoori A. et al. 2015. "Obesity and Pro12Ala polymorphism of peroxisome proliferator-activated receptor-gamma gene in healthy adults: A systematic review and meta-analysis." *Ann. Nutr. Metab.* 67(2): 104–118.

Moghaddami K. et al. 2018. "The effect of interval training intensity on protein levels of ATGL and Perilpin-5 in visceral adipose tissue of type 2 diabetic male rats." *Internat. J. Appl. Exer. Physiol.* 7(4): 62–70.

Mori H. et al. 2001. "Ala substitution in PPAR-γ is associated with resistance to development of diabetes in the general population and possible involvement in impairment of insulin secretion in individuals with type 2 diabetes." *Diabetes* 50(4): 891–894.

Motta V. et al. 2016. "High-intensity interval training (swimming) significantly improves the adverse metabolism and comorbidities in diet-induced obese mice." *J. Sports Med. Phys. Fitness* 56(5): 655–663.

Osawa H. et al. 2009. "PPARgamma Pro12Ala Pro/Pro and resistin SNP-420 G/G genotypes are synergistically associated with plasma resistin in the Japanese general population." *Clin. Endocrinol. (Oxf).* 71(3): 341–345.

Regieli J.J. et al. 2009. "PPAR gamma variant influences angiographic outcome and 10-year cardiovascular risk in male symptomatic coronary artery disease patients." *Diabetes Care* 32(5): 839–844.

Ruchat S.M. et al. 2010. "Improvements in glucose homeostasis in response to regular exercise are influenced by the PPARG Pro12Ala variant: Results from the HERITAGE Family Study." *Diabetologia* 53(4): 679–689.

Stumvoll M. et al. 2002. "The peroxisome proliferator-activated receptor-γ2 Pro12Ala polymorphism." *Diabetes* 51(8): 2341–2347.

Tyagi S. et al. 2011. "The peroxisome proliferator-activated receptor: A family of nuclear receptors role in various diseases." *J. Adv. Pharm. Technol. Res.* 2(4): 236–240.

Vidal-Puig A. et al. 1996. "Peroxisome proliferator-activated receptor gene expression in human tissues: Effects of obesity, weight loss, and regulation by insulin and glucocorticoids." *J. Clin. Invest.* 97: 2553-2561.

Wang S. et al. 2015. "Resveratrol induces brown-like adipocyte formation in white fat through activation of AMP-activated protein kinase (AMPK) α1." *Int. J. Obes. (Lond)* 39(6): 967–976.

Background for APOA2

Basiri M. et al. 2015. "APOA2 −256T>C polymorphism interacts with saturated fatty acids intake to affect anthropometric and hormonal variables in type 2 diabetic patients." *Genes Nutr.* 10(3): 15.

Corella D. et al. 2007. "The -256T>C polymorphism in the apolipoprotein A-II gene promoter is associated with body mass index and food intake in the genetics of lipid lowering drugs and diet network study." *Clin. Chem.* 53(60): 1144–1152.

Dolores C. et al. 2009. "APOA2, dietary fat and body mass index: Replication of a gene-diet interaction in three independent populations." *Arch. Intern. Med.* 169(20): 1897–1906.

Noorshahi N. et al. 2016. "APOA II genotypes frequency and their interaction with saturated fatty acids consumption on lipid profile of patients with type 2 diabetes." *Clin. Nutr.* 35(4): 907–911.

Ruotolo G. et al. 2001. "Human evidence that the apolipoprotein A-II gene is implicated in visceral fat accumulation and metabolism of triglyceride-rich lipoproteins." *Circulation* 104: 1223–1228.

Smith C. et al 2012. "Apolipoprotein A-II polymorphism: Relationships to behavioural and hormonal mediators of obesity." *Int. J. Obes. (Lond)* 36(1): 130–136.

Xiao J. et al. 2008. "The apolipoprotein AII rs5082 variant is associated with reduced risk of coronary artery disease in an Australian male population." *Atherosclerosis* 199(2): 333–339.

Zaki M. et al. 2013. "APOA2 polymorphism in relation to obesity and lipid metabolism." *Cholesterol* Epub. 289481.

Background for FABP2

Baier L. and Hanson R. 2004. "Genetic studies of the aetiology of type 2 diabetes in Pima Indians." *Diabetes* 53(5): 1181–1186.

Baier L. et al. 1995. "An amino acid substitution in the human intestinal fatty acid binding protein is associated with increased fatty acid binding, increased fat oxidation, and insulin resistance." *J. Clin. Invest.* 95(3): 1281–1287.

Boden G. et al. 1995. "Effects of a 48-h fat infusion on insulin secretion and glucose utilization." *Diabetes* 44(10): 1239–1242.

Carlsson M. et al. 2000. "The T 54 allele of the intestinal fatty acid-binding protein 2 is associated with a parental history of stroke." *J. Clin. Endocrinol. Metab.* 85(8): 2801–2804.

Chamberlain A. et al. 2009. "Ala54Thr polymorphism of the fatty acid binding protein 2 gene and saturated fat intake in relation to lipid levels and insulin resistance: The Coronary Artery Risk Development in Young Adults (CARDIA) study." *Metabolism* 58(9): 1222–1228.

Chiu K.C. et al. 2001. "The A54T polymorphism at the intestinal fatty acid binding protein 2 is associated with insulin resistance in glucose tolerant Caucasians." *BMC Genet.* 2: 7.

Formanack M. and Baier L. 2004. "Variation in the FABP2 promoter affects gene expression: Implications for prior association studies." *Diabetologia* 47(2): 349–351.

Hegele R. et al. 1996. "Genetic variation of intestinal fatty acid-binding protein associated with variation in body mass in aboriginal Canadians." *J. Clin. Endocrinol. Metabol.* 81(12): 4334–4338.

Kalhan S.C. 2009. "Fatty acids, insulin resistance, and protein metabolism." *J. Clin. Endocrinol. Metab.* 94(8): 2725–2727.

Knowles W. et al. 1978. "Diabetes incidence and prevalence in Pima Indians: A 19-fold greater incidence than in Rochester, Minnesota." *Am. J. Epidemiol.* 108(6): 497–505.

Liu Y. et al. 2015. "Association of the FABP2 Ala54Thr polymorphism with type 2 diabetes, obesity, and metabolic syndrome: A population-based case-control study and a systematic meta-analysis." *Genet. Mol. Res.* 14(1): 1155–1168.

Martinez-Lopez E. et al. 2013. "Effect of Ala54Thr polymorphism of FABP2 on anthropometric and biochemical variables in response to a moderate-fat diet." *Nutrition* 29(1): 46–51.

Qiu C.-J. et al. "Association between FABP2 Ala54Thr polymorphisms and type 2 diabetes mellitus risk: A huge review and meta-analysis." *J. Cell. Mol. Med.* 18(12): 2530–2535.

Schulz L. et al. 2015. "High risk populations: The Pima Indians of Arizona and Mexico." *Curr. Obes. Rep.* 4(1): 92–98.

Sears B. et al. 2015. "The role of fatty acids in insulin resistance." *Lipids Health Dis.* 14: 121.

Xu L. et al. 2016. (original article in Chinese) "Effect of FABP2 gene G54A polymorphism on lipid and glucose metabolism in simple obesity children." *Wei Sheng Yan Jiu* 45(1): 1–7.

Yamada K. et al. 1997. "Association between Ala54Thr substitution of the fatty acid-binding protein 2 gene with insulin resistance and intra-abdominal fat thickness in Japanese men." *Diabetologia* 40(6): 706–710.

Background for TCF7L2

Corella D. et al. 2013. "Mediterranean diet reduces the adverse effect of the *TCF7L2*-rs7903146 polymorphism on cardiovascular risk factors and stroke incidence: A randomized controlled trial in a high-cardiovascular-risk population." *Diabetes Care* 36(11): 3803–3811.

Folsom A. et al. 2008. "Variation in TCF7L2 and increased risk of colon cancer: The atherosclerosis risk in communities (ARIC) study." *Diabetes Care* 31(5): 905–909.

Freathy R.M. et al. 2007. "Type 2 diabetes TCF7L2 risk genotypes alter birth weight: A study of 24,053 individuals." *Am. J. Hum. Genet.* 80: 1150–1161.

Grant S.F. et al. 2006. "Variant of transcription factor 7-like 2 (TCF7L2) gene confers risk of type 2 diabetes." *Nat. Genet.* 38(3): 320–323.

Hindy G. et al. 2012. "Role of *TCF7L2* risk variant and dietary fibre intake on incident type 2 diabetes." *Diabetologia* 55(10): 2646–2654.

Korner A. et al. 2007. "TCF7L2 gene polymorphisms confer an increased risk for early impairment of glucose metabolism and increased height in obese children." *J. Clin. Endocrinol. Metab.* 92(5): 1956–1960.

Lyssenko V. et al. 2007. "Mechanisms by which common variants in the TCF7L2 gene increase risk of type 2 diabetes." *J. Clin. Invest.* 117(8): 2155–2163.

Ouhaibi-Djellouli H. et al. 2014. "The *TCF7L2* rs7903146 polymorphism, dietary intakes and type 2 diabetes risk in an Algerian population." *BMC Genetics* 15: Article Number 134.

Phillips C.M. et al. 2012. "Dietary saturated fat, gender and genetic variation at the TCF7L2 locus predict the development of metabolic syndrome." *J. Nutr. Biochem.* 23(3): 239–244.

Sousa A.G. et al. 2009. "TCF7L2 polymorphism rs7903146 is associated with coronary artery disease severity and mortality." *PLOS One* 4(11): 7697.

Tong Y. et al. 2009. "Association between TCF7L2 gene polymorphisms and susceptibility to type 2 Diabetes Mellitus: A large Human Genome Epidemiology (HuGE) review and meta-analysis." *BMC Med. Genet.* 10: 15.

Van de Wetering M. et al. 2002. "The beta-catenin/TCF-4 complex imposes a crypt progenitor phenotype on colorectal cancer cells." *Cell* 111(2): 241–250.

Welcome Trust Case Control Consortium. 2007. "Genome-wide association study of 14,000 cases of seven common diseases and 3,000 shared controls." *Nature* 447(7145): 661–678.

Wong N.A. et al. 2002. "Beta-catenin - a linchpin in colorectal carcinogenesis?" *Am. J. Pathol.* 160(2): 389–401.

Background for IRS1

Alharbi K.K. et al. 2014. "Association of the genetic variants of insulin receptor substrate 1 (IRS1) with type 2 diabetes mellitus in a Saudi population." *Endocrine* 47(2): 472–477.

Ericson U. et al. 2013. "Sex-specific interactions between the IRS1 polymorphism and intakes of carbohydrates and fat on incident type 2 diabetes." *Am. J. Clin. Nutr.* 97(1): 208–216.

Hirbal M.L. et al. 2000. "The Gly972Arg amino acid polymorphism in IRS1 affects glucose metabolism in skeletal muscle cells." *J. Clin. Endocrinol. Metab.* 85(5): 2004–2013.

Kalaany N.Y. et al. 2009. "Tumours with PI3K activation are resistant to dietary restriction." *Nature* 458(7239): 725–731.

Kilpelainen T.O. et al. 2011. "Genetic variation near IRS1 associates with reduced adiposity and an impaired metabolic profile." *Nat. Genet.* 43(8): 753–760.

Maglio C. et al. 2013. "The IRS1 rs2943641 variant and risk of future cancer among morbidly obese individuals." *J. Clin. Endocrinol. Metab.* 98(4): E785–789.

Mahmutovic L. et al. 2019. "Association of IRS1 genetic variants with glucose control and insulin resistance in type 2 diabetic patients from Bosnia and Herzegovina." *Drug. Metab. Pers. Ther.* Volume 34: Issue 1.

Ohshige T. et al. 2011 "Association of new loci identified in European genome-wide association studies with susceptibility to type 2 diabetes in the Japanese." *PLOS One* 6(10): 26911.

Qi Q. et al. 2011. "Insulin receptor substrate 1 gene variation modifies insulin resistance response to weight-loss diets in a 2-year randomized trial: The Preventing Overweight Using Novel Dietary Strategies (POUNDS LOST) trial." *Circulation* 124(5): 563–571.

Rung J. et al. 2009. "Genetic variant near IRS1 is associated with type 2 diabetes, insulin resistance and hyperinsulinemia." *Nat. Genet.* 41(10): 1110–1115.

Sharma R. et al. 2011. "The type 2 diabetes and insulin-resistance locus near IRS1 is a determinant of HDL cholesterol and triglycerides levels among diabetic subjects." *Atherosclerosis* 216(1): 157–160.

Soyal S. et al. 2015. "Associations of haplotypes upstream of IRS1 with insulin resistance, type 2 diabetes, dyslipidemia, preclinical atherosclerosis, and skeletal muscle LOC646736 mRNA levels." *J.Diab. Res.* Article ID 405371.

Thirone A.C. et al. 2006. "Tissue-specific roles of IRS proteins in insulin signalling and glucose transport." *Trends Enocrinol. Metab.* 17(2): 72–78.

Yiannakouris N. et al. 2012. "IRS1 gene variants, dysglycaemic metabolic changes and type 2 diabetes risk." *Nutr. Metab. Cardiovasc. Dis.* 22(12): 1024–1030.

Zheng J. et al. 2013. "Modulation by dietary fat and carbohydrate of IRS1 association with type 2 diabetes traits in two populations of different ancestries." *Diabetes Care* 36(9): 2621–2627.

Background for Stress Genes

De Oliveira C. et al. 2011. "High-fat diet and glucocorticoid treatment cause hyperglycemia associated with adiponectin receptor alteration." *Lipids in Health and Disease* 10: 11.

Dias B. et al. 2014. "Parental olfactory experience influences behavior and neural structure in subsequent generations." *Nature Neuroscience* 17: 89–96.

Dusek J.A et al. 2008. "Genomic counter-stress changes induced by the relaxation response." *PLOS One* 3(7): e2576.

Park S. et al. 2016. "Interactions with the MC4R rs17782313 variant, mental stress and energy intake and the risk of obesity in Genome Epidemiology Study." *Nutrition & Metabolism* 13: 38.

Powell N.D. et al. 2013. "Social stress up-regulates inflammatory gene expression in the leukocyte transcriptome via β-adrenergic induction of myelopoiesis." *Proc. Natl. Acad. Sci. U.S.A.* 110(41): 16574-16579.

Roy S. et al. 2005. "Wound site neutrophil transcription in response to psychological stress in young men." *Gene Expression* 12(4–6): 273–287.

Yehuda R. et al. 2016. "Holocaust exposure induced intergenerational effects on FKBP5 methylation." *Biol. Psych.* 80(5): 372–380.

Background for ADRB2

Augusto A. et al. 2010. "Very important pharmocogen summary of ADRB2." *Pharmacogenet. Genomics* 20(1): 64–69.

Bea J. et al. 2010. "Lifestyle modifies the relationship between body composition and adrenergic receptor genetic polymorphisms, *ADRB2*,

ADRB3 and *ADRA2B*: A secondary analysis of a randomized controlled trial of physical activity among postmenopausal women." *Behav. Genet.* 40(5): 10.

Daghestani M.H. et al. 2010. "The Gln27Glu Polymorphism in β2-Adrenergic receptor gene is linked to hypertriglyceridemia, hyperinsulinemia and hyperLeptinemia in Saudis." *Lipids Health Dis.* 9:90

Ishiyama-Shigemoto S. et al. 1999. "Association of polymorphisms in the beta 2-adrenergic receptor gene with obesity, hypertriglyceridaemia, and diabetes mellitus." *Diabetologia* 42(1): 98–101.

Jocken J.W and Blaak E.E. 2008. "Catecholamine-induced lipolysis in adipose tissue and skeletal muscle in obesity." *Physiol. Behav.* 94(2): 219–230.

Large V. et al. 1997. "Human beta-2 adrenoceptor gene polymorphisms are highly frequent in obesity and associate with altered adipocyte beta-2 adrenoceptor function." *J. Clin. Invest.* 100(12): 3005–3013.

Lima J. et al. 2007. "Association analyses of adrenergic polymorphisms with obesity and other metabolic alterations." *Metabolism* 56(6): 757–765.

Martinez J.A. et al. 2003. "Obesity risk is associated with carbohydrate intake in women carrying the Gln27Glu beta2-adrenoceptor polymorphism." *J. Nutri.* 133(8): 2549–2554.

Masouo K. and Lambert G.W. 2011. "Relationships of adrenoceptor polymorphisms with obesity." *J. Obes.* 2011: e609485.

Rebecca M. et al. 2015. "Neurogenetic variations in norepinephrine availability enhance perceptual vividness." *J. Neurosci.* 35(16): 6506–6516.

Ruiz J. et al. 2012. "Role of $β_2$-adrenergic receptor polymorphisms on body weight and body composition response to energy restriction in obese women: Preliminary results." *Obesity* 19(1): 212–215.

Saliba L. et al. 2014. "Obesity-related gene *ADRB2*, *ADRB3* and *GHR* polymorphisms and the response to a weight loss diet intervention in adult women." *Genet. Mol. Bio.* 37(1): 15–22.

Szendrei B. et al. 2016. "Influence of ADRB2 Gln27Glu and ADRB3 Trp64Arg polymorphisms on body weight and body composition changes after a controlled weight-loss intervention." *Appl. Physiol. Nutr. Metab.* 41(3): 307–314.

Todd R. et al. 2015. "Neurogenetic variations in norepinephrine availability enhance perceptual vividness." *J. Neurosci.* 35(16): 6506–6516.

Xie W. 2018. "ADRA2B deletion variant and enhanced cognitive processing of emotional information: A meta-analytical review." *Neurosci. Biobehav. Rev.* 92: 402–416.

Background for NR3C2

Bogdan R. et al. 2010. "The impact of mineralocorticoid receptor ISO/VAL genotype (rs5522) and stress on reward learning." *Genes Brain Behav.* 9(6): 658–667.

Bogdan R. et al. 2012. "Mineralocorticoid receptor Iso/Val (rs5522) genotype moderates the association between previous childhood emotional neglect and amygdala reactivity." *Am. J. Psych.* 169(5): 515–522.

DeRijk R. and de Kloet E.R. 2005. "Corticosteroid receptor genetic polymorphisms and stress responsivity." *Endocrine* 28(3): 263-270.

Durand G. 2018. "Influence of allelic variations in relation to norepinephrine and mineralocorticoid receptors on psychopathic traits: A pilot study. *Peer J.* 6: e4528.

Emad S. et al. 1991. "Overexpression and characterization of the human mineralocorticoid receptor." *J. Biolog.Chem.* 266(27): 18072–18081.

Kortmann G.L. et al. 2012. "The role of mineralocorticoid receptor gene function polymorphism in the symptom dimensions of persistent ADHD." *Eur. Arch. Psychiatry Clin. Neurosci.* 26(3): 181–188.

Martinez F. et al. 2009. "Association of a mineralocorticoid receptor gene polymorphism with hypertension in a Spanish population." *Am. J. Hypertens.* 22(6): 649–655.

McEwen B.S. 2004. "Protection and damage from acute and chronic stress: Allostasis and allostatic overload and relevance to the pathophysiology of psychiatric disorders." *Ann. N.Y. Acad. Sci.* 1032: 1–7.

Muller M.B. et al. 2003. "Limbic corticotropin-releasing hormone receptor 1 mediates anxiety-related behavior and hormonal adaptation to stress." *Nat. Neurosci.* 6(10): 1100–1107.

Roel H. et al. 2006. "A common polymorphism in the mineralocorticoid receptor modulates stress responsiveness."*J.Clin. Endocrinol. Metab.* 91(12): 5083–5089.

Slof-Op't Landt M.C. et al. 2014. "A common mineralocorticoid receptor polymorphism (I180V) interacts with life events in relation to perfectionism in eating disorders: A pilot study." *Eur. Eat. Disord. Rev.* 22(6): 423–429.

ter Heegde F. et al. 2015. "The brain mineralocorticoid receptor and stress resilience." *Psychoneuroendocrinology* 52: 92–110.

Van Leeuwen N. et al. 2011. "Human mineralocorticoid receptor (MR) gene haplotypes modulate MR expression and transactivation: Implication for the stress response." *Psychoneuroendocrinology* 36(5): 699–709.

Background for CRCH1

Cicchetti D. and Rogosch F. 2014. "Genetic moderation of child maltreatment effects on depression and internalizing symptoms by serotonin transporter linked polymorphic region (5-HTTLPR), brain-derived nerve factor (BDNF) and corticotropin releasing hormone receptor 1 (CRHR1) genes in African American children." *Devel. Psychopath.* 26(4): 1219–1239.

Contoreggi C. et al. 2004. "Nonpeptide corticotropin-releasing hormone receptor type 1 antagonists and their applications in psychosomatic disorders." *Neuroendocrinology* 80(2): 111–123.

Gilespie C.F. et al. 2009. "Risk and resilience: Genetic and environmental influences on development of the stress response." *Depress. Anxiety* 26(11): 984–992.

Licino J. et al. 2004. "Association of cortiocohormone releasing receptor 1 haplotype and antidepressant treatment response." *Mol. Psychiatry* 9(12): 1075–1082.

Licino J. et al. 2019. "CRHR1- corticotropin releasing hormone receptor 1 Homo sapiens." *Wikigenes gene review.* www.wikigenes.org/e/gene/e/1394.html.

Muller M.B. et al. 2003. "Limbic corticotropin-releasing hormone receptor 1 mediates anxiety-related behavior and hormonal adaptation to stress." *Nat. Neurosci.* 6(10): 1100–1107.

Schartner C. et al. 2017. "CRHR1 promoter hypomethylation: An epigenetic readout of panic disorder?" *Eur. Neuropsychopharmacol.* 27(4): 360–371.

Schmid B. et al. 2010. "Interacting effects of *CRHR1* gene and stressful life events on drinking initiation and progression among 19-year-olds." Int. J. Neuropsychopharmacology 13(6) 703–714.

Selfdecode. 2019. "CRHR1 (Corticotropin releasing hormone receptor 1)." (https://www.selfdecode.com/gene/crhr1/)

Background for FKBP5

Binder E.B. 2009. "The role of FKBP5, a co-chaperone of the glucocorticoid receptor in the pathogenesis and therapy of affective and anxiety disorders." *Psychoneuroendocrinology* 34(1): 186–195.

Bryant R.A. et al. 2016. "Association of FKBP5 polymorphisms and resting-state activity in a frontotemporal-parietal network." *Transl. Psychiatry* 6(10): e925.

Denny W.B. et al. 2000. "Squirrel monkey immunophilin FKBP51 is a potent inhibitor of glucocorticoid receptor binding." *Endocrinology* 141: 4107–4113.

Gillespie C.F. et al. 2009. "Risk and resilience: Genetic and environmental influences on development of the stress response." *Depress. Anxiety* 26(11): 984–992.

Hartmann I.B. et al. 2016. "The FKBP5 polymorphism rs1360780 is associated with lower weight loss after bariatric surgery: 26 months of follow-up." *Surg. Obes. Relat. Dis.* 12(8): 1554–1560.

Hubler T.R. et al. 2004. "Intronic hormone response elements mediate regulation of FKBP5 by progestins and glucocorticoids." *Cell Stress Chaperones* 9(3): 243–252.

Linnstaedt S.D. et al. 2018. "A functional riboSNitch in the 3'UTR of FKBP5 alters microRNA-320a binding efficiency and mediates vulnerability to chronic posttraumatic pain." *J. Neurosci.* 38(39): 8407–8420.

Luijik M.P. et al. 2010. "FKBP5 and resistant attachment predict cortisol reactivity in infants: Gene-environment interaction." *Psychoneuroendocrinology* 35(10): 1454–1461.

Wilker S. et al. 2014. "The role of FKBP5 genotype in moderating long-term effectiveness of exposure-based psychotherapy for posttraumatic stress disorder." *Transl. Psych.* 4: 403.

Wochnik G.M. et al. 2005. "FK506-binding proteins 51 and 52 differentially regulate dynein interaction and nuclear translocation of the glucocorticoid receptor in mammalian cells." *J. Biol. Chem.* 280(6): 4609–4616.

Yang L. et al. 2012. "Hypothalamic Fkbp51 is induced by fasting, and elevated hypothalamic expression promotes obese phenotypes." *Am. J. Physiol. Endocrinol. Metab.* 302(8): E987–E991.

Zannas A. et al. 2016. "Gene–Stress–Epigenetic regulation of *FKBP5*: Clinical and translational implications." *Neuropsychopharmacoly* 41(1): 261–274.

Background for Nutrients and Meal Timing

Barnosky A.R. et al. 2014. "Intermittent fasting vs. daily calorie restriction for type 2 diabetes prevention: A review of human findings." *Transl. Res.* 164(4): 302–311.

Chamberlain A. et al. 2009. "Ala54Thr polymorphism of the fatty acid binding protein 2 gene and saturated fat intake in relation to lipid levels and insulin resistance: The Coronary Artery Risk Development in Young Adults (CARDIA) study." *Metabolism* 58(9): 1222–1228.

Giovannucci E. et al. 2016. "Association of animal and plant protein intake with all-cause and cause-specific mortality." *JAMA Int. Med.* 176(10): 1453–1463.

Goodrick C.L. et al. 1983. "Differential effects of intermittent feeding and voluntary exercise on body weight and lifespan in adult rats." *J. Gerontol.* 38(1): 36–45.

Heibronn L. et al. 2005. "Glucose tolerance and skeletal muscle gene expression in response to alternate day fasting." *Obes. Res.* 13(3): 574–581.

Hjort L. et al. 2017. "36 h fasting of young men influences adipose tissue DNA methylation of *LEP* and *ADIPOQ* in a birth weight-dependent manner." *Clin. Epigenetics* 9: 40.

Levine M.E. et al. 2014. *"Low protein intake is associated with a major reduction in IGF1, cancer and overall mortality in the 65 and younger but not older population."* Cell Metab. 19(3): 407–417.

Martin B. et al. 2006. "Caloric restriction and intermittent fasting: Two potential diets for successful brain aging." *Ageing Res. Rev.* 5(3): 332–353.

Rothschild J. et al. 2014. "Time-restricted feeding and risk of metabolic disease: A review of human and animal studies". *Nutr. Rev.* 72(5): 308–318.

Sartorius K. et al. 2018. "Does high-carbohydrate intake lead to increased risk of obesity? A systematic review and meta-analysis." *BMJ Open.* 8(2): e018449.

Stockman M.C. et al. 2018. "Intermittent fasting: Is the wait worth the weight?" *Curr. Obes. Rep.* 7(2): 172–185.

Zhu Y. et al. 2013. "Metabolic regulation of Sirtuins upon fasting and the implication for cancer." *Curr. Opin. Oncol.* 25(6): 630–636.

Background for Supplements

TMC

Chatterjee A. et al. 2010. "Efficacy of a natural weight management herbal formulation in obese human subjects. LOWAT." *51st Annual Meeting, American College of Nutrition*, New York, NY, Oct 7–9, 2010. Abstract 53, 29(5): 518.

Dasgupta N. and De B. 2004. "Antioxidant activity of *Piper betle* leaf extract in vitro." *Food Chemistry* 88(2): 219–224.

Giancaterini A. et al. 2000. "Acetyl-L- Carnitine infusion increases glucose disposal in type 2 diabetes patients." *Metabolism* 49(6): 704–708.

Iossa S. et al. 2002. "Acetyl-L-Carntine supplementation differently influences nutrient partitioning, serum Leptin concentration and skeletal muscle mitochondrial respiration in young and old rats." *J. Nutr.* 132(4): 636–642.

Sengupta K. et al. 2012. "Efficacy of an herbal formulation LI10903F containing *Dolichos biflorus* and *Piper betle* extracts on weight management." *Lipids Health Dis.* 11: 176.

Van Weyenberg S. et al. 2009. "Increased plasma Leptin through l-carnitine supplementation is associated with an enhanced glucose tolerance in healthy ponies." *J. Anim. Physiol. Anim. Nutr. (Berl)* 93(2): 203–208.

Sereniten Plus

Adzemovic M.Z. et al. 2013. "Efficacy of vitamin D in treating multiple sclerosis-like neuroinflammation depends on developmental stage." *Exp. Neurol.* 249: 39–48.

Guesdon B. et al. 2006. "A tryptic hydrolysate from bovine milk alpha-S1-casein improves sleep in rats subjected to chronic mild stress." *Peptides* 27(6): 1476–1482.

Juneja L.R. et al. 1999. "L-theanine: A unique amino acid of green tea and its relaxation effect in humans." *Trends Food Sci. Tech.* 10: 199–204.

Kim J.H. et al. 2007. "Efficacy of alpha-S1-casein hydrolysate on stress-related symptoms in women." *Eur. J. Clin. Nutr.* 61(4): 536–541.

Kimura K. et al. 2007. "Anti-Stress, behavioural and magnetoencephalography effects of an l-theanine-based nutrient drink: A randomised, double-blind, placebo-controlled, crossover trial." *Biol. Psych.* (serial online) 74(1): 39–45.

Messaoudi M. et al. 2005. "Effects of a tryptic hydrolysate from bovine milk alpha-S1-casein on hemodynamic responses in healthy human volunteers facing successive mental and physical stress situations." *Eur. J. Nutr.* 44(2): 128–132.

Miclo L. et al. 2001. "Characterization of alpha-casozepine, a tryptic peptide from bovine alpha(s1)-casein with benzodiazepine-like activity." *FASEB J.* 15(10): 1780–1782.

Prietl B.T. et al. 2013. "Vitamin D and immune function." *Nutrients* 5(7): 2502–2521.

Metabolic Xtra

Sun C. et al. 2007. "SIRT1 improves insulin sensitivity under insulin-resistant conditions by repressing PTP1B." *Cell Metab.* 6(4): 307–319.

Resveratrol Extra

Wang S. et al. 2015. "Resveratrol induces brown-like adipocyte formation in white fat through activation of AMP-activated protein kinase (AMPK) α1." *Int. J. Obesity* 39(6): 967–976.

DopaPlus

Stansnley B.J. et al. 2013. "L-dopa-induced dopamine synthesis and oxidative stress in serotonergic cells." *Neuropharmacol.* 67: 243–251.

Young S.N. 2007. "L-Tyrosine to alleviate the effects of stress?" *J. Psychiatry Neurosci.* 32(3): 224.

Whey Satisfied

Birketvedt G.S. et al. 2005. "Experiences with three different fiber supplements." *Med. Sci. Monit.* 11(1): 15–18.

Jung E. et al. 2017. "Low-dose yeast hydrolysate in treatment of obesity and weight loss." *Preventive Nutrition and Food Science.* 22(1):45–49.

Rao T.P. 2016. "Role of guar fiber in appetite control." *Physiol. & Behav.* 164(A): 277–283.

Veldhorst A. et al. 2008. "Protein-induced satiety: Effects and mechanisms of different proteins." *Physiology & Behavior* 94(2): 300–307.

Vita P.M. et al. 1992. "Chronic use of glucomannan in the dietary treatment of severe obesity." *Minerva. Med.* 83(3): 135–139.

Walsh D.E. et al. 1984. "Effect of glucomannan on obese patients: A clinical study." *Int. J. Obes.* 8(4): 289–293.

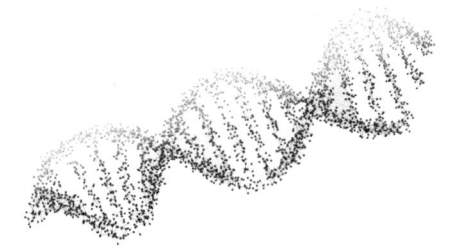

ABOUT THE AUTHORS

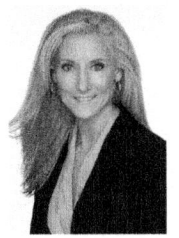

Dr. Penny Kendall-Reed BSc ND
Penny is a Naturopathic Doctor with a clinical practise in Toronto, Canada. She travels worldwide lecturing on genetics and the interpretation and treatment of single nucleotide polymorphisms (SNPs) relating to metabolic and neuroendocrine disorders. She is the creator of the integrated genetics platform GeneRx.ca and is a member of the scientific board for PureGenomics. She is a medical consultant for Douglas Laboratories and Pure Encapsulations.

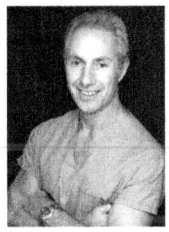

Dr. Stephen Reed BM BCh MA(Oxford) MSc(Toronto) FRCSC
Stephen is a staff orthopaedic surgeon at the Humber River Hospital in Toronto, Canada. He shares an interest in the role genetics plays in the disease process and the integration of traditional and naturopathic medicine to improve patient outcome.

We are a husband and wife team who believe in the complementary value of traditional and naturopathic medicine. We have co-authored a number of books exploring the synergy of these fields in achieving optimum patient care.

OTHER BOOKS

The New Naturopathic Diet (Winding Star Press, 2002, ISBN: 1 55082 302 7)

The No Crave Diet (Virgin Books, 2008, ISBN: 978 0 7535 1313 2)

The Complete Doctor's Stress Solution (Robert Rose Inc. 2004, ISBN 0 7788 0096 2)

Healing Arthritis (Quarry Press Inc. 2002, ISBN 1 55082 312 4)

The Complete Doctor's Healthy Back Bible (Robert Rose Inc. 2004, ISBN 0 7788 0091 1)

Printed in Great Britain
by Amazon